Aloe
Isn't
Medicine,
and Yet...
It Cures!

Father Romano Zago, OFM
(Order of Friars Minor)

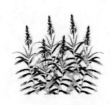

Also by Father Romano Zago

Cancer Can Be Cured
Includes :The Scientific Monographic History of Aloe
Vera and Aloe Arborescens

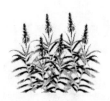

Disclaimer Notice:

The information, scientific studies, specific phytotherapeutic solutions, and opinions discussed in this book, while carefully researched, are offered for educational purposes only about a natural remedy for different illnesses. They are not intended as medical advice nor intended to diagnose or treat any individual's health problems. You should not discontinue any course of health treatment or undertake any new treatment without consulting your healthcare practitioner of choice. Neither the publisher, author nor any other person who is directly or indirectly related to this publication dispenses medical advice, nor do they prescribe any remedies or assume any responsibility for those who choose to treat themselves.

Legal Notice: The health-related statements in this book have not been evaluated by the U. S. Food and Drug Administration.

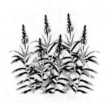

Contents

Letter of presentation 1

Preface..3

Part I: Variations In My Recipe 5

Introduction 7

Father Romano Zago's recipe......................................11

Questions and Answers 15

Weights and measurements 15

Using pure Aloe 17

The gathering of the leaves....................................19

The presence of water in the Aloe leaves 21

Honey in the case of diabetes................................23

Alcohol in the case of alcoholism 24

Various types of Aloe 26

A meter of Aloe leaves 28

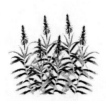

Part II: Reasons for Using the Preparation 31

    Introduction 33

    Aloe is not toxic 33

    Natural Aloe vs. commercial Aloe 38

    Aloe is nourishment 40

    Aloe strengthens the immune system 43

    Aloe as a preventive measure 44

    Aloe as a cure 46

    Phenomena or reactions in your body 50

    The body's excretion path 52

Part III: The Use of Aloe for the Cure of Illnesses 57

Introduction 59

Afterward 133

Bibliography 135

Glossary 165

Index 179

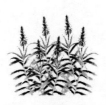

Letter Of Presentation

At the time of the first edition of the Brazilian original of **Aloe Isn't Medicine, and Yet...It Cures!**, I sent a copy to my friend Cardinal Lorscheider, Archbishop of Aparecida, Sao Paulo, Brazil. His Eminence, very kindly and of his own volition, replied with the letter that I will transcribe and which, as a Letter of Presentation, can appropriately illustrate the existing Italian translation.

Aparecida, Sao Paulo, 2 Jan. 2003

Dearest Fr. Romano Zago

I am writing to send you my best wishes for your new book: **Aloe Isn't Medicine, and Yet...It Cures!** Best wishes!

I read the book from beginning to end. I liked it very much. From the author's dedication – you have a beautiful handwriting – to the conclusion, I experienced a whole lot of joy reading it. You are able to maintain a colloquial style from beginning to end. A very simple, pleasant and happy style. You speak with the reader. This way you are successful in keeping the attention of whoever intends to follow you throughout the work. He who starts reading it finds himself compelled to finish it.

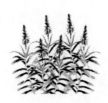

The difference with the first book is substantial, although the essence is the same. It is a book destined to do a lot of good. This book is extraordinary, even at a spiritual level. You can be proud of it. The front cover is very nice as well.

Having read your book, I can conclude that you live a happy and joyous life. I feel this very deeply; you transmit your jovial and optimistic ways very clearly. Once again, my best wishes!

Dearest Father Romano, keep on being always full of vitality and enthusiasm. May the good Lord bless you and keep you under His protection. I hope that you are very happy.

Your friend,

Luigi Cardinal Lorscheider

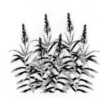

Preface

Dedicating myself to the present task, I kept foremost in my mind the state of my fellow Brazilian citizens who, according to recent statistics and to our great dismay, live on the threshold of poverty in one of the richest countries in the world in terms of natural resources. Fifty million people, almost one third of the country's total population, are poor and without sustenance. These people cannot afford the luxury of having a health plan – nor even think of it – not even in their wildest dreams! Public health is in a very deep state of degradation. Professionals, poorly compensated by the Single Health System (SUS), offer very unreliable medical assistance. Patients pile up at queues from early morning, wait for an appointment for a visit or for a consultation they will have months later. Chances are that they end up dying in hospital corridors well before then. Remedies, always adjusted in price before inflation, turn out to be prohibitive for these patients. It is for these fellow patriots that I am writing this book. It is my main intent to offer help and support to my poor for their sufferings. Forgive me if I express my thoughts, but it is the only way I know to stay at peace with my conscience. Yes, it is little, I know, but it is all that I have learned to do.

If this book is successful in helping reduce even a small percentage of the sufferings and in contributing to an improvement of my brothers' medical and financial situation, for me this will be reason for happiness and commemoration.

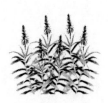

Four years after being printed in Brazil (2002)[1], **Aloe Isn't Medicine, and Yet...It Cures!,** Italian and English translations are available, so the Brazilian reality, by way of Italy, reaches the developed world. I desire that the benefits from Aloe, which the Brazilians have attained, may be enjoyed by people like yourselves, who have the means of treating your health.

In return I ask the IMF and the G7 powers to cancel, or at least suspend for a period of five to ten years, interests applied to the Brazilian Foreign Debt, so that such an astronomical sum of money, a bleeding wound for my country, may be channelled towards providing basic necessities such as education, housing, health, public safety, and transportation (hydro-road-rail). Within five years, we will be able to walk on our own legs. It is my wish that this one-third of the population may enjoy the bare minimum of dignity a human being deserves. In exchange, you will have the benefits from having Aloe at your disposal.

The Author

[1]ZAGO, Romano. **Aloe Isn't Medicine, and Yet...It Cures!** Petrópolis, RJ: Vozes, 2002 (1st edition).

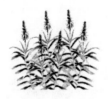

Part I

Variations In My Recipe

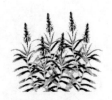

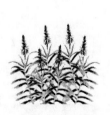

Introduction

The human body heals itself from within and, because of its more than 300 phytotherapeutic substances, the juice from the whole leaf of Aloe arborescens plant provides the perfect complement to the biological requirements of the body. In Aloe arborescens, you will find a true arsenal of useful substances important and essential for maintaining healthy cell functioning, such as monosaccharide oils, polysaccharides, anthraquinones, terpenoids, enzymes, proteins, amino acids, metals, minerals, vitamins, etc. The cleansing performed with the recipe of Aloe arborescens, honey and distillate detoxifies the body, renews the blood and strengthens the immune system so the body can restore itself to health. People have used the Brazilian plant recipe to provide the body's immune system a potent remedy for over 100 types of illnesses, including cancer, diabetes, depression and obesity.

Those who have read **Cancer Can Be Cured!**, the first book by Father Romano Zago, have found themselves facing some challenging decisions. We have learned of this through written correspondence, telephone calls, faxes, and e-mails regarding the home recipe of Aloe, honey and distillate (see **Cancer Can Be Cured!**, chapter *The Recipe*). People have gotten lost in details of little importance, some of which have created obstacles to preparation of the product. Details are important, but not to the point of causing confusion. As a Dutch saying has it: "One cannot see the forest for the trees."

In this first part, we get back to the main theme in a succession of questions and answers in an attempt to provide clarification so you may navigate safely in these waters. That way, you will feel free to prepare the product.

In the body of the book **Cancer Can Be Cured!**, for at least fifteen pages, we present the Aloe, honey and distillate-based recipe. We are not all the same, which is a good thing! On the contrary, since no person is the same as another, we find it appropriate to present all the possible variations.

Before we get into the details, we think it is essential to point out that the recipe is not static, as someone might deduce in reading the book. On the contrary, it is dynamic and flexible, as long as the personal health conditions of those who look to it are respected.

The ingredients are the same: Aloe (in whole leaf form), honey and distillate. In the book, we must present some prototypes, but they must not be taken as standards. Please personalize according to your imagination and needs. If you act freely, there is no need to set rigid rules. With time and practice, you will determine the amounts according to weight or measurement, as many others have done before you, ever since the recipe was made public.

One thing is to navigate in open waters for the first time and another – quite different – is the job of the expert seaman. It is so for every human activity. After a practice period, one does it automatically. It will be that way when you make your preparation.

Let's start by commenting on a few practical points. Our objective is that you make the best use of freedom granted by God to his children.

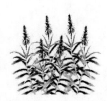

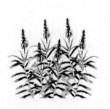

Father Romano Zago's Recipe

Ingredients*

- **350 grams (.77 lbs.) of Aloe arborescens leaves,** two or three or four or five, whatever may be necessary to achieve the correct weight.

- **Half a kilo (1.1 lbs.) of bees' honey** (organic honey)

- **40-50 ml (about 8 tsps.) of** distillate (grappa, cognac, whiskey, etc.)

*1 kilogram = 1,000 grams; 1 lb. = 455 grams. A commercially made equivalent comes in a 16-oz. violite bottle.

Preparation

Using a dry piece of cloth or sponge, remove the thorns from the edges of the leaves and the dust that may have collected on them. Cut the leaves into pieces (without removing the skin) and put them in a blender, together with the honey and the chosen distillate. Blend well. The mix is ready for consumption. It must not be strained or cooked and it must be refrigerated in a dark, well-sealed jar.

Recommended Doses

Take **one** tablespoon 20 to 30 minutes **before each of the three main meals** (breakfast, lunch, and supper). Shake well

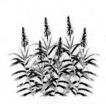

before use. Once you have started this treatment, it is important to finish the entire jar. As soon as the treatment is completed, a medical check-up is recommended (especially if we are dealing with a cancer case). The results of the blood analysis will give an indication of its effectiveness, and this will suggest the procedures to follow thereafter. If the results indicate that there hasn't been an improvement with the first jar, it is necessary to repeat the procedure after a 5- to 10-day interval.

Repeat this procedure as many times as necessary to cure the illness. If one has not achieved the desired results after four full treatments, the dose must be doubled – that is, two tablespoons before each meal.

I have learned from the many letters I have received that many readers of this book cannot possibly prepare the juice recipe from home for various reasons and must rely on a commercial source for this 10-day liquid recipe supplied in a 16-oz. dark bottle. In this case, it is important to choose a manufacturer that uses premium quality five-year-old Aloe arborescens plants harvested at the proper time, processed by grinding the whole leaf into a juice without heating, cold pressing or freeze drying in order to retain all the active poly-saccharides and phytonutrients needed to guarantee maximum effectiveness. Finally, the recipe needs to be stabilized for a long shelf life without the use of harmful preservatives.

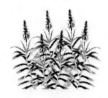

"This miraculous preparation truly is the unending hand of Providence for the hopeless!" – Sister Maria Angiolina

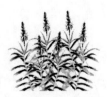

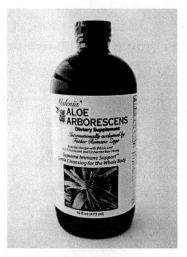

Commercial production of the Aloe Arborescens Brazilian Recipe for supreme immune support is manufactured in North America and in Europe as a dietary supplement and distributed by health professionals and health product distributors.

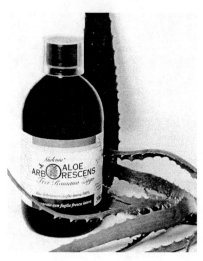

For more information on

the Brazilian immune formula and the scientific papers and research abstracts on the properties of this aloe species, go to aloearborescens.org.

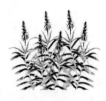

Questions and Answers

1. Weights and measurements

Question: The universal recipe calls for 500 grams of honey (1.1 lbs.), Aloe arborescens and distillate. Must it be exactly 500 grams (1.1 lbs)? Couldn't it be a little more or a little less?

Answer: So that it may give some benefits, the treatment should last at least ten days. If one were to go over ten days, it wouldn't matter. Finish the contents of the jar without leaving any residue. If it lasts 10, 15, or 20 days, it is equally all right. Finish the contents of the jar, independent of the duration.

With time and practice, you will determine if you need 500 grams of honey (1.1 lbs.) or if, for example, 300 grams (.66 lbs.) might be enough to complete the ten-day cycle. You could argue that it isn't worth debating over one hundred or two hundred grams of honey. I agree. But, in these difficult times, if you can save a little, why not do so? It is with one kernel of wheat at a time that the chicken fills up its crop, states a wise proverb.

Speaking of honey, it is clear that it will always be you who leads the show. Let's imagine that you prepared the product using the ingredients according to the universal recipe. But your son, for whom it is intended, being used to sweets, finds it unpalatable. He complains. You can avoid a conflict. Solve the

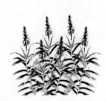

problem: add more honey. You can do this without reducing the quantity of Aloe. The important aspect is that your child gets the Aloe, and that he does so independently of the quantity or of the mathematical accuracy. If you are able to find a solution to the health problem afflicting your son without having reduced the quantity of Aloe, consider yourself a winner.

Now, let's imagine the opposite. You have a liver problem. The liver is not receptive to sweets. If you keep the ingredients called for in the universal recipe, it is possible that your intestines will have contractions when you ingest the preparation. Try inverting the figures. If the recipe calls for 300 grams of Aloe and 500 grams of honey, then switch the two. Use 300 grams of honey and 500 grams of Aloe. You may be surprised to find out that your liver will not react like an untameable horse as it did before when you used the amounts called for in the universal recipe. And how wonderful if you are able to solve your liver problem in such an economical and side effect-free way!

Now, have you understood why the recipe is dynamic and not static? The figures in the recipe are only relative, as in the Far East. We Westerners look at formulas in a mathematical way: $2 + 2 = 4$, whereas for the Orientals, yes $2 + 2 = 4$ as well, but for them, it can also be 5 or 3. Do not worry so much about mathematical accuracy, since life is rich and generous. Learn from it. Let yourself be led by what it suggests or asks. And live!

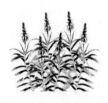

2. Using pure Aloe

Question: Is it possible to use pure Aloe, that is, without the honey and the distillate?

Answer: One could ask himself yet another question, as a final clarification: What are the functions of the honey and the distillate in the base Aloe recipe?

First of all, let's make it clear that we could use Aloe all by itself, that is, without the honey or the distillate. I repeat, we could.

The honey and the distillate stimulate the abundant active principles present in the plant, improving its effectiveness on the illness.

Aloe could be used by itself – pure – if you really wanted to. Know, though, that Aloe stimulated by honey and distillate may give better results. In other words, do not leave out these other ingredients unless you have good reasons to do so.

Honey is used because, since ancient times, it has been considered an excellent genuine food with many qualities. Honey is able to move to all parts of the body – the remote corners. It is the vehicle that carries the Aloe, which cleanses and removes the impurities it finds along the way. This procedure performs general cleansing of the entire body – especially the blood – and can heal cancer and other correlated

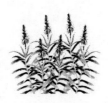

diseases, such as rheumatism, arthrosis, etc. Everyone knows blood is vital to the human body.

Distillate on its own may seem the least important ingredient. The first explanation I received on the importance of using distillate was that in far-off places, in caves where there is still no electricity, people don't have fridges. Without this appliance, the product could go bad. Distillate is used to preserve the preparation, preventing it from perishing. This is a plausible explanation.

Later I heard an odd although pertinent reason: the distillate is used to dilate the blood vessels. To clarify this, I was given an explanation of this function with reference to clinical cases. When a patient has circulation problems, he is prescribed a dose of whisky to try to correct this deficiency. This explanation seems logical and the example has provided me with a better understanding of the function of the distillate. It also became clear that, in older people especially, dilated blood vessels would speed up the cleansing action of the Aloe and honey.

Later I learned the true function of the distillate from scientific research. The third component of the preparation is not used by chance or whim. The explanation is that when the Aloe leaf is cut, it gives off a viscous, stringy, bitter, greenish liquid rich in properties called aloin. The human body is unable to absorb this fully if it is not dissolved in the distillate.

I wish to stress that the first two explanations are not without sense. The first makes us understand that the blend can

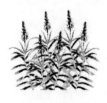

also be kept out of the fridge without going bad, in the cupboard or dresser, as long as it is away from light. The second points out the vasodilator function of the distillate.

With regard to distilled drinks, it must be mentioned that the following are all equally effective: Brazilian grappa (cachaca), cognac or whisky, Mexican tequila, Italian grappa, Dutch bols, araq from Palestine and other Arab countries, and others. Neither wine nor beer must be used, as they are fermented, with lower concentrations of alcohol. If necessary, they have to be used in greater quantities. No kinds of liqueur must be used, as these are sugar-based products. It amounts to about 1% of the recipe or what you would find in a cough formula.

3. The gathering of the leaves

Question: Are there instructions for the gathering of the leaves?

Answer: Concerning the gathering of the leaves that will be used to make the home preparation, do not use small leaves (leaf buds), or dried or yellow leaves (the Japanese, aware of the preciousness of the plant, use even the dried or yellow leaves, just so as not to waste them).

Use only the fully developed adult leaves. This is only natural. In nature, everything happens according to specific laws. An orange or a tangerine, as big as a little finger, is complete. But, to be able to eat them, one needs to wait until they ripen. The two-year-old girl and the ninety-year-old woman are two full-bodied women, but unable to conceive, and so on. Everything has its time. Nature will point out the moment of maturity. One must have patience and wait. And, when they're ripe, the leaves can be harvested.

It is important to know that the Aloe plant is active at night and "dormant" during the day. That is, it becomes "totally impermeable, hermetically closing all its stomas during the day." In other words, being a desert plant, it keeps its pores closed during the day to avoid the evaporation of water due to heat, and opens them at night to gather the morning dew.

With this in mind, pick the raw material (the leaves) either before sunrise or after sunset.

Avoid preparing the recipe under the direct rays of either natural or artificial light. The effect of sun rays or artificial lighting is to reduce the plant's active principles against tumors. Avoid rays. This is the reason the jar should be protected from light. In commercial production, a 16-oz. dark violite colored bottle is used. This bottle is proven to block light between 450-700 mm, the range known to damage nutrients.

By the way, aren't these the proper precautions taken when transporting such products as wine and beer – fermented beverages – from their production sites to the consumption sites? Dark containers are used. We resort to such expedients so that rays of sunlight do not alter the quality of the product

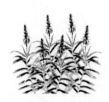

during transportation. As you can see, every detail has logic to it, bringing us a pinch of wisdom.

4. The presence of water in the Aloe leaves

Question: What about rain? What if I want to wash the leaves?

Answer: A lot of people run into problems making the Aloe preparation on account of the rain and their excessive zeal in cleaning the leaves.

Yes, they can be washed, if you are a scrupulous person when it comes to hygiene. I respect that very much.

As far as rain is concerned, in winter, the rainiest time of the year, get your umbrella and rain boots and, protected from the elements as you are, go into the garden where you have that magnificent Aloe specimen and pick, let's say, 50 grams worth of leaves. Combine with 100 grams of honey, one tablespoon of the distillate of your choice and make this first batch of the preparation as if it were the entire preparation. Such quantity will last more or less three days. Having used up this first batch, immediately create, without a break, a second batch. Continue doing this until you have finished the treatment, which must last a minimum of 10 days (if it lasts a day or two longer, better yet). And let it rain…

By preparing it in stages, you will avoid the risk of oxidation, which is always a danger when our raw material is

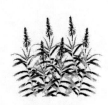

inebriated with water. The Aloe leaf absorbs water easily because of its spongy nature. The plant, being a desert plant, knows that in its natural habitat it rains very little. It has learned that it is vital to store the precious liquid. An intelligent plant!

Now, your preparation – free of preservatives, prepared with leaves picked after a rainfall, or washed – is destined to oxidize. This is the same process that meat undergoes when not frozen – it deteriorates. Similarly, an apple becomes dark only a few minutes after it has been cut, compromising the quality of the product.

Preparing it in stages ensures the freshness of the product and practically eliminates the possibility of oxidation.

Note: The presence of water makes the product oxidize more rapidly. Nothing more. But even with this higher water content, the Aloe's medicinal properties don't decrease in the least. The only drawback lies in the fact that, without preservatives, the high quantity of water predisposes your product to oxidation, because water is not a good preservative. However, it will maintain its medicinal properties. Therefore, the drier the leaves the less likely that your home preparation may oxidize.

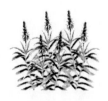

5. Honey in the case of diabetes

Question: How does the honey in the recipe affect diabetics?

Answer: It is fundamental to know that Aloe cures diabetes. Yes, I repeat, Aloe, by itself, has cured diabetes. Who makes this claim? American publications do. Check Bibliography for references to studies.

In your case, use pure Aloe, meaning all by itself, with or without distillate. But since it is bitter (and it has to be!), when you take it, have some freshly made fruit, vegetable, or legume juice ready so you can neutralize the bitter taste immediately.

Note: Regarding honey, if it is genuine, meaning made by bees, not man-made, it won't be bad for diabetics, because honey made by bees does not undergo a refining process. Refined honey is considered unhealthy for the system: sugar, salt, flour, rice, oil, etc. If honey is authentic, it will never be harmful to users, least of all to diabetics.

If, on the other hand, you are not in favor of honey, eliminate it from your recipe. Eliminate it if you are convinced you cannot have anything sweet. Honey is sweet, so honey for you is forbidden.

How come?

Logical. The mind gives orders to the body. Say you are convinced a diabetic cannot have honey because it is sweet, and if you use it, your blood sugars will be high. Here is the subjective phenomenon that controls or has an effect on what is objective.

Do not despair for this limitation. With or without honey, Aloe acts beneficially for your system; it may not be at 100 percent, so accept 70 or 40 percent. But do not deprive yourself of it.

Aloe has cured people of diabetes. Why not try it? You could be one of them. Go ahead; experience this benefit all the way.

6. Alcohol in the case of alcoholism

Question: How should one proceed in the case of a reformed alcoholic?

Answer: Are you undergoing treatment with Alcoholics Anonymous (AA) to cure yourself of this addiction? If even a single drop of alcohol could take you back to your former condition, taking you once again to the bottom of the well, run away from this drink like the devil from the cross. Do not play with fire. Stay well clear of using the alcoholic ingredient called for in the recipe. Use only Aloe and honey. Will it give only partial benefits? Yes, but it's fine. It's much better to do that than to risk going back to that old horror. Aloe and honey are perfectly tolerable. They don't constitute a problem.

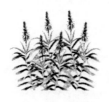

If, however, you decide to take Aloe by itself and you find it too bitter, turn to the juice method described regarding the use of honey for the diabetic.

But if you are a person who doesn't give up easily, take a deep breath and swallow that juice, even though it is bitter. Let it do its job. It knows what it has to do. Wait for the benefits. The results won't be long in coming.

Speaking of alcoholics, it is worth noting that Aloe acts as a detoxifier and, as such, reduces the desire for alcohol. It does the same thing for addiction to smoking and drugs. Combined with a strong willpower, addicts realize it is possible to control themselves.

The frantic search for alcohol could depend not only on some form of deception on behalf of the person who makes use of it, but it could also originate from some kind of physical necessity: the system needs something it lacks, in this case, zinc. The patient looks for a solution to the problem, drinking alcoholic beverages, because in them he finds the substance he lacks.

A simple way to remedy a system zinc deficiency would be to stop by a pharmacy and ask for a mix of multivitamin and mineral salts rich in zinc. Since Aloe contains zinc, there have been cases in which people have reduced their need for tobacco, alcohol and drugs. If the symptoms do not disappear, consult a doctor.

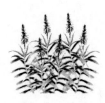

7. Various types of Aloe

Question: Which type of Aloe should I choose among the many different types in existence?

Answer: There are those who have difficulty choosing one type of Aloe because of the many different types in existence. In **Cancer Can Be Cured!**, we recommend using Aloe arborescens in your homemade preparation. Aloe arborescens presents a lower quantity of gel; you can use this type of Aloe without making use of preservatives for conservation and without risk that the product will oxidize easily.

But let's suppose you have only Aloe vera Barbadensis Miller in your garden. Do not despair. As far as its medicinal properties are concerned, this type of Aloe is equally good. The only disadvantage is that Aloe vera Barbadensis Miller is very rich in gel, a very desirable quality at the commercial market level where major corporations focus on maximizing their profits.

Commercial marketers erroneously claim that the plant's medicinal properties are present only in the gel. What deception! The gel is water, my friend. About 95% of it is water. Did you know that? During long rainy periods, it could even reach as much as 99%. It would not be true to say that the gel is worthless. However, it would be just as erroneous to say that the gel is the only important part. Gel is luxury-filtered water, but it's still water.

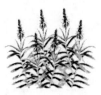

Now, with such high water content, you can understand why the homemade preparation, in which there is no room for preservatives, tends to oxidize quickly. How can you resolve this problem? Given that it is undesirable to make use of preservatives (they are carcinogenic!), the answer is simple: peel the leaf as you would an orange to reduce the volume of the pulp or that of the crystalline gel that is found inside it. When you have obtained approximately 300 grams (.77 lbs.) of skin (leaf), add the honey and the distillate and grind everything. As you can see, in terms of volume, you have obtained more or less an equal amount to what you would have obtained had you used Aloe arborescens.

About the leftover gel, do not throw it out. The gel is precious! You can use it externally on your entire body, from the top of your head to the bottom of your feet. Due to the active principle lignin, very abundant in Aloe, your skin will appreciate it, becoming velvety, moisturized and rejuvenated.

Besides its direct application on the skin, put any leftover gel in a jar with alcohol. The day you come down with any kind of muscle ailments, you will have at your immediate disposal an excellent remedy to massage lightly over the painful area.

From a medicinal viewpoint, these two types of Aloes are similar. We must learn how to deal with the gel. That brings us back to the problem of excessive water. The less water the homemade preparation contains, the longer it will last without oxidizing.

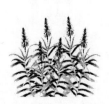

As expected, having to abide by rigid stability criteria, the commercial product will not present oxidation problems.

8. A meter (3.3 ft.) of Aloe leaves

Question: Measure or weigh?

Answer: In **Cancer Can Be Cured!**, we recommend a meter (3.3 ft.) of leaves, combined with honey and the distillate, to make your homemade preparation. People have quickly realized that, using Aloe arborescens, they obtain a specific volume inside the jar, but using Aloe vera barbadensis, they get a greater volume, almost twice as much. A meter (3.3 ft.) of leaves of the Aloe vera barbadensis variety yields at least twice the volume of the final preparation using the same amount of leaves of the arborescens variety (a variety explained in our book). Do not be surprised by this; it is perfectly understandable.

From Italy, we get the following suggestion: in place of measurement-meter, use weight-grams. How many grams? About 300 grams (.77 lbs.). This is a valid suggestion because 300 grams of barbadensis and 300 grams of arborescens will always be 300 grams (.77 lbs.).

In the case of linear measurements, you can come up with a one-meter quantity either by increasing or decreasing the number of leaves according to your personal requirements, so you can come up with the 300 grams (.77 lbs.) quantity called for by the recipe or go above that value by adding more Aloe if you so desire, in case you use weight as a form of measure. Follow your own instincts, slowly getting away from weights and measurements. Use your common sense. The important thing is balance. This is only a suggestion. At first, follow the measurements called for in the universal recipe and, as you gain practical experience, you may opt to modify the amounts according to your personal requirements. It is up to you.

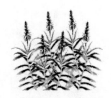

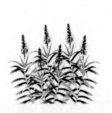

Part II

Reasons For Using The Preparation

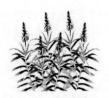

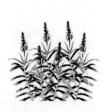

Introduction

In this second part, we present some specifics that we must never lose sight of when dealing with the Aloe plant, known in Brazil under the name of Babosa, a plant that grows very well in your garden. (The fact that you have taken the initiative to grow this plant is a demonstration that you are an intelligent person). Do not lose sight of these points. Be aware of them when you make the preparation, either as a preventive measure or as a cure. Keep the following in mind:

- Aloe is not toxic
- Natural Aloe vs. commercial Aloe
- Aloe is nourishment
- Aloe strengthens the immune system
- Aloe as a preventive measure
- Aloe as a cure
- Aloe and the body's reaction to it
- Aloe and the body's excretion paths

Aloe is not toxic

In the **Cancer Can Be Cured!** chapter "Is Aloe toxic?", we deal with this subject, turning to the authors of two great works: **A Silent Cure**, by Bill C. Coats and Robert Ahola, and **Aloe: Myth-Magic-Medicine**, by Odus M. Hennessee and Bill R.

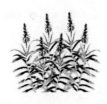

Cook, quoting the pages of the respective works of the two notable authors.

Despite this, there are rumors that Aloe is poisonous, especially when taken continuously and in large quantities.

Our answer, based on more than 20 years of experience, is that the Aloe plant in your garden will never be poisonous. You can reply: "That which is positively affirmed may be positive or negative." I will explain later. On February 25, 2000, the National Health Vigilance Agency, a body of the Ministry of Health in Brazil, published RDC Resolution No. 17 dated 24-02-2000 that approves the technical regulation of the registry of phytotherapeutic medicine. In the appendix of this resolution, there is a list of thirteen different plants, including Aloe, whose consumption does not produce negative side effects.

At this point, you may argue that this refers exclusively to a topical use of the plant. Here's my answer.

In 1999, I traveled across Brazil giving more than 200 lectures (please note that there are only 365 days in a year) in auditoriums, not to mention radio and television programs. In 2000, I gave 150 lectures. In these meetings, 50% of the listeners stated they were familiar with Aloe, saying they had taken it orally in the doses called for in our recipe. Not a single voice was heard saying that our preparation, taken orally, had any negative effects on the user. It could very well be that it didn't always bring about a cure for all who used it. We wish! Imagine if it were so! But it didn't harm anyone.

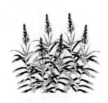

Regarding the quantity, you can attest to the fact that, in **Cancer Can Be Cured!**, we have never stated that you may take Aloe in large quantities, by the ton. What does "large quantities" mean?

Yes, we agree that abusing or going overboard with quantity can be harmful, but this is true of all aspects of human activity. Water, too, in excess, kills. Take a flood, for instance. There is no need to look very far to substantiate these truths.

As far as taking Aloe continuously, in **Cancer Can Be Cured!** we have never made this assertion. We suggest you take a break after each jar. We have always recommended taking a break between each complete preparation.

There are many people who make use of Aloe 365 days a year on their own initiative. These people affirm that this hasn't had any ill effects on them whatsoever. They use it every day because they feel it gives them an excellent quality of life, allowing them to do away with the need for any type of allopathic remedy.

In short, following the recommended dosage, you may make use of Aloe any time you consider it necessary, with or without a break between complete preparations.

An excess of aloin, one of the substances found in Aloe, may be poisonous. Commercial marketers of this substance obtain it from Aloe through an extraction process and sell it through pharmacies in powder, crystal or tablet forms. If you abuse this

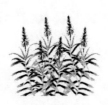

processed Aloe, you could have unpleasant consequences, but this is valid for the extract of any plant.

Why, then, has the notion that Aloe is toxic spread so freely? Where does it originate? I wish I could believe that the people who spread this notion actually believe it themselves. In other words, why don't they provide proof for it?

Generally, it is argued that aloin, when taken in large quantities, is responsible for the toxicity problem. But in our case, if you follow our instructions, you will never risk being poisoned because the daily quantity of aloin taken will always be minimal. It would be just like arguing that you can't drink coffee because it contains caffeine. Caffeine is only one of the many substances present in coffee, a useful product for the body. Problems could be caused by an excessive use of this product – 80 cups of coffee a day, for instance.

My concern is that the real motive behind the spreading of this notion is the commercial marketers' attempt to promote "other interests," such as being able to claim that their products are free of aloin, a toxic substance.

I stress that aloin acts synergistically in the body, meaning that all the substances in the plant are released and work in complete unison, like the instruments of an orchestra. The body absorbs what it needs and, activating all of its mechanisms, eliminates what it already has enough of. So why wouldn't it need some percentage of aloin?

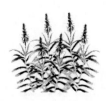

By the way, staying on the subject, aloin is also present in drugs for rheumatism. Couldn't the body be suffering, to a small degree, from this ailment? Suddenly, with the consumption of this product, it could rid itself of this condition. I repeat, the body knows what it needs.

Remember: Aloin is toxic only when consumed in large quantities and in concentrated form, meaning that the raw material has been subjected to high temperatures. Our recipe proposes using the Aloe you have in your garden, free of poisonous chemicals, naturally grown and taken in sensible amounts. Such preparation will never harm you. On the contrary, Aloe will only have beneficial effects on you.

You see, at times I think the problem is greed. The home preparation costs you little or nothing. The commercial product, on the other hand, costs money. The expense of the home recipe is insignificant in comparison with the commercial product. However, the results obtained with the home recipe are similar to those obtained with the commercial product. It could be that the multi-nationals do not take this very kindly since they are interested in selling their products.

I hope that one day I will be able to inform you of the exact correspondence between Aloe and aloin (how many grams of Aloe are necessary to produce a gram of aloin?), and how many grams of aloin your body can tolerate without harm. I would like to find a laboratory that will do this for the consumers of the Brazilian preparation so all consumers can be assured that

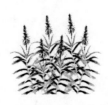

the presence of aloin does not harm them. It takes a good dose of common sense to deal with this misinformation sensibly, for it does nothing but confuse inexperienced and uninformed consumers.

Natural Aloe vs. Commercial Aloe

Generally, the assertion that Aloe is poisonous is generated by commercial marketers and supported by laboratories and even by encyclopedias used as sources of research. What is the truth?

It can be toxic if taken in large quantities. Aloe, obtained through a process that subjects it to high temperatures, such as distillation, followed by crystallization or pulverization, and consumed in large quantities, will undoubtedly compromise one's health, as we have seen in the preceding chapter.

This phenomenon doesn't pertain solely to Aloe, but to all plants. Even lettuce or tea, subjected to high temperatures, may be toxic up to a point. Aloe is no exception. Such data is supplied to us by homeopathy, a therapeutic method that consists of prescribing a patient, in a very diluted and dynamic form, a substance capable of producing similar effects as those presented by him. **Note:** This method was created by Dr. Samuel Hahnemann (1755-1843) at the end of the eighteenth century (Dizionario Houaiss da Lingua Portuguesa. Rio de Janeiro: Editora Objetiva Ltda, 2001, p.1546). The homeopathic substances are obtained through a pharmaceutical maceration process in 192 proof alcohol for a specified period of time, and given as treatment in the form of drops, mixed with water and never prescribed in heavy doses, given its concentration.

In the meantime, if you use the leaves of your own Aloe plant, grown in your own garden, your natural plant is completely safe. We have never recommended that anyone use it excessively. When you first start taking it, we recommend you begin with a tablespoon's worth (10 ml) each morning, a second tablespoon at noon, and a third at supper time. This is the recommended dose for an adult. If we are dealing with children, the dose is proportional to their ages. Double the quantity to two tablespoons' worth three times a day only after you have consumed two or three jars without the desired results. On the fourth jar, if you are still not cured, you can increase it to three tablespoons three times a day, and so on.

However, if you notice something wrong, and you suspect that it may have to do with the preparation, reduce the quantity. Increasing the quantity gradually, you will be able to perform this verification without harming yourself.

Note: If you only have access to Aloe in its concentrated form, have a pharmacist or a chemist guide you so that, through his expertise, he may suggest the recommended dose expected to cure your ailment without unwarranted risks due to unintentional overdose. In any case, your plant will always supply you with the right leaves for constant use, without negative side effects.

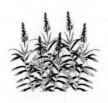

Aloe is Nourishment

It is fundamental to keep in mind Aloe's abundant supply of medicinal properties, known to man as far back as ancient times. As a result, it presents itself more as a nourishing supplement than as medicine. If you decide to take Aloe, know that you have opted for an alternative that is complete nourishment. There are those who, after getting used to taking this preparation of Aloe, honey and distillate, skip breakfast in the morning without any loss of energy.

In Aloe, you will find a true arsenal of useful substances, important and essential for the body, such as enzymes, vitamins, proteins, amino acids, metals, minerals, mono-saccharide oils, polysaccharides, etc.

The German pharmacopoeia, in the 1873 edition during Bismarck's time, already included more than 300 pharma-ceutical substances present in Aloe. Today, modern literature confirms this with list after list of such substances as the result of honest laboratory research objectively seeking the truth.

It's a curious thing that many ill-informed people state that Aloe does not have any medicinal substances. In my view, we are either dealing with a case of such gross ignorance that it precludes the acceptance of the curative effects of plants in general (there is a science, known as **phytotherapy**, that deals with the treatment and prevention of diseases through plant

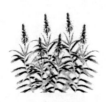

use), or such "scientists" manipulate the instruments in their "laboratory," forcing them to yield pre-conceived results. With such analysis in hand, they contact the mass media, which thrives on sensationalism, and declare that they haven't recorded any therapeutic phenomenon worthy of note. Even worse, they can even claim that the Aloe plant does not contain any active ingredients. Uninformed readers or listeners, not having access to a laboratory, accept such truth and abandon the wonderful opportunity to turn to a simple, economical and effective treatment because they have been deprived of real scientific support. If those who worked in a laboratory showed just minimum honesty, the results today concerning Aloe would be known to the entire world. If people argue that such a laboratory has recorded nothing about the active principles of the plant, they don't have much to stand on, as they didn't perform the analyses. Such a laboratory should be considered a second or third grade laboratory, because such scientists per-form science, keeping in mind other interests – their own! – and not scientific results. Science is performed when one searches for truth above all else. But, as we know, sooner or later, the naked truth will come out, whether one likes it or not. It is for this reason that the Gospel states: Truth will save you (John 8,32).

In the 1960s, foreign scientists disguised as missionaries belonging to some church met with our Amazonian natives and deceitfully gained their phytotherapeutic knowledge.

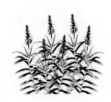

Beginning with the 1980s, true scientists have been carrying away our flora, transforming into medicine the active components of our plants. Example? The Japanese classified the *spina santa* and produced half a dozen remedies from it. Note that the spina santa does not grow in Japan; the Japanese come here to obtain the raw material.

Likewise with mushrooms. The book by Takashi Mizzuno (see Bibliography) presents fungo Agaricus as a 99.4% effective inhibitor of tumors.

Even the stone splitter has been proven to actually split stones, as it has always been known to our ancestors. It corrodes, continuously scratching the kidney stone, until it is small enough to come out through the normal excretion ducts.

And then there is the anona tree, which destroys cancer 10,000 times more effectively than chemotherapy without side effects. May the Americans enjoy it!

Lately, German and French scientists have classified the picão and the carurù as herbs with curative properties. The Germans, not long ago, classified the rapadura (the scraper), a tablet of unprocessed sugar, produced centuries ago by the inhabitants of northeastern Brazil.

This bio-piracy, the illegitimate appropriation and illegal trafficking of live material, goes on without restraint in Brazil.

A good thing is that, in today's magazines, newspapers, and on television, there is more evidence that scientists agree on the

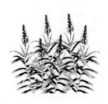

existence of medicinal plants. The existence of these plants has been studied and accepted by the scientific media and adopted by numerous orthodox medicine professionals.

Aloe strengthens the immune system

Aloe's more than 300 phytotherapeutic substances and its active components strengthen the immune system, predisposing the body to confront the most difficult hardships it may encounter during life. That is why we have heard testimonials such as the following by people who have made use of it:

"I always used to come down with colds and coughs. I used to get sick three or four times a year. Getting sick was routine. Now, ever since I have been taking Aloe, I haven't caught one cold... Good-bye, cold!"

What did this person do? Simple. Turning to the Aloe recipe, he strengthened his defenses. And you, with your defenses up, will no longer catch colds or AIDS, just to mention two extremes. It's when you have a weak immune system that you are exposed to all types of illnesses. To give a football example, a team with a solid defense is unlikely to be scored upon, but if the defense is weak, it will be scored upon many times. It is this way in everything. The same goes for health matters. Therefore, get yourself ready; practice prevention. Or, as the simple people wisely say, it is better to prevent than it is to cure.

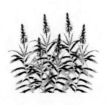

Taking Aloe, you will be ready for anything. If the storm is approaching, you already know where to take shelter.

Summarizing, if you take Aloe, you will be investing in the best health plan, which will repay you with an excellent quality of life, without large expenses.

Aloe as a preventive measure

The preparation, either as a preventive measure or as a curative treatment, is always the same. What changes is the interval between jars. In the preventive treatment, it is the user who determines the length of the interval.

Let's say you are enjoying enviable health. You sleep well. You eat well.

Nothing is bothering you. You don't even know what a headache or stomach ache is. You work. You don't need to diet. You attribute this healthy picture to your moderation; you do not overindulge in anything.

No excesses! is your life's motto. I ask: can a person in such good health take Aloe?

Yes, he can. So long as he wants to.

How many times a year? Once? Three times? Five times?

As many times as he likes. There are no rules that regulate taking Aloe as a preventive cure.

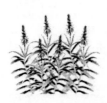

How many jars a year can one take?

He could take one jar a year. Or he could take one every six months. Or one every three months. Or one every two months. Or one a month. The individual decides. Treat it as if it were orange juice, rich in vitamin C. How many times a year can we take orange juice? As much as we like! There are no rules or criteria that determine how many times a year we can take orange juice.

We must emphasize that taking Aloe does not compromise one's health. On the contrary. Not only will your health be maintained but it will even be improved. You will experience an overall well being. You will realize it.

Reader, please allow me to give a suggestion to my senior friends. Even though you may be a person up in years, but in good health, I suggest you take Aloe often during a year. Why? Simple. As the years pile on, we lose substances the body is incapable of replenishing as easily as it used to. Here, then, is the aging process: we lose substances the body does not know how to replenish. Aloe, so rich in substances, will slow down this natural process by replenishing a good bit of the mineral salts, vitamins, enzymes, proteins, etc. so vital to maintaining good health. Surely such a procedure will reward you with an improved quality of life and better health.

How gratifying it is to reach full maturity without sclerosis, with good eyesight and hearing, able to get about freely, fully in control of your faculties, aware, lucid, entertaining dreams and

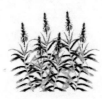

making plans for life! How much of the Aloe cure should you take a year? Take one jar. When its contents are used up, schedule yourself for a second treatment in one to two months. For a younger person, the time interval between jars may be greater.

It's not a matter of snubbing beauty or declaring the discovery of the fountain of youth. (By the way, it is not a sin to look young and beautiful.) Why not look mature and also beautiful, showing fewer years than what your birth certificate says? In the end, the essential thing is the quality of life. If you can live to age 150, then may it be in good health. Quality of life, certainly, will guarantee long life. Let's work at it.

Aloe as a cure

As we said in the preceding chapter, the difference between preventive and curative treatments lies in the interval between jars. The preparation is the same. You are the one who determines that interval between jars.

In the curative treatment, the shorter this interval the better – three or four days or one week at the most. The point is that you should never give disease a rest so it can regroup. If your prognosis is not promising, you can start with a continuous treatment, without breaks. Keep taking the preparation until you have achieved a complete recovery, a condition that must be monitored through appropriate medical examinations, preferably with the doctor who first diagnosed your illness. If the medical analysis demonstrates that the illness has not been completely defeated, continue with the treatment without long intervals between jars. Bear in mind that if you are shooting for a complete healing, the shorter the interval between jars the better. Continue with the treatment until you achieve your goal, which is healing, increasing the dose if necessary.

Theoretically, it will give results. I say theoretically because, in practice, full cooperation on the part of the individual is necessary. Unfortunately, many times this factor is missing. Without this cooperation, healing becomes much more difficult to achieve. When the patient cooperates with his healing, therapies perform "miracles," producing results well beyond expectations.

It is important to remember that human beings are the essence of a number of factors: body, spirit, mind, sensibility, intelligence, feelings, and emotions. Such factors are inter-connected. If one of them isn't well, the others also suffer in one form or another. The job of the individual is to make sure all factors are balanced. It is the negative side of a human being. As such, illness does not necessarily arise from a physical ailment. It can have its root cause in the psychological or spiritual or mental side. This is why it is fundamental to maintain health at all levels, in perfect balance. When this balance is present, health prospects are better. Illnesses enter and exit holistically. Do not forget that illness, such as pain and fever, is the body's alarm signal, telling you that something of an aggressive,

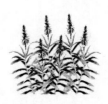

dangerous nature is springing up. It is an alarm bell; find out its cause.

The procedure of allopathic medicine is to treat with drugs, to eliminate the pain without finding out the cause. In the case of a stuck auto horn blowing, the most comfortable course of action is to disconnect the electric wires. A very easy task, but do not be surprised if two miles down the road the engine melts. A headache? A stomach ache? Try to understand the cause.

It is generally acknowledged that official medicine is very effective against pain, but shouldn't it be similarly effective at determining the cause of pain? Ideal situation: know the origin of both the pain and the illness; the problem must be resolved at the roots. Look for the means to eliminate it there.

The majority of people use Aloe as a **curative measure.** It would be much more important to use it as a **preventive measure.** Aloe is a very powerful detoxifier. As such, it can cure because it restores the cells and the body. Proof of this can be found in the factual testimonials of a number of people, locals as well as from other parts of the world who, following a colostomy (colon surgery) brought on by an intestinal obstruction, took several jars of our preparation. As a result, their affected organs regained their normal functioning to the point that they were able to eliminate the uncomfortable bag they had been fitted with at the time of surgery and that they were destined to keep for the rest of their lives.

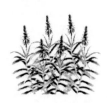

It is undeniable that Aloe, because of its extraordinary and powerful curative properties, is the most sought-after option for consumers. **However, we cannot overemphasize that this preparation should be sought for its preventive powers.**

Aloe can be an exceptional detoxifier. Use Aloe's therapeutic qualities to free yourself of the illnesses afflicting you.

It shouldn't be necessary to say that you are the principal guardian of your health. You should be familiar with the right amount of anything for yourself, and what you can and can't do. You should eat a balanced, rational diet, without chemical toxins, and without alcohol, smoking and drug abuse. You are in charge of the show. Your doctor can only do so much if you don't cooperate. You are the first line of defense for yourself. It is you who should be most interested in your well being. Take care of your health and you will live happily. Without good health, everything else – money, power, honors – is worth little or nothing. How much pleasure would life give you in the absence of good health? Pay more attention to nutritional value rather than taste or appetite. It's a measure of prudence. People say wisely: Fish dies through the mouth. Likewise for man, I add.

Today, official medicine accepts as a fact that man is a machine created by God to last approximately up to 150 years with good health. What happens to the remaining 50% or more of life for the majority of us mortals?

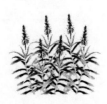

Let's imagine a truck carrying soybeans in kernel form from its production region to the port of Rio Grande about 1,000 kilometers away. It so happens that the vehicle has a hidden hole in its body. During the trip, with all the bouncing due to the irregularities of the road surface, a large amount of the product is lost, to the joy of a number of little animals that find sustenance and are able to continue to live and multiply.

Through the course of life, we lose days, weeks, years of it – losses that, with small measures, could easily be avoided. Until we apply corrective measures (it would only take a plug to eliminate that hole in the body of the truck), we are forced to use the nutritional savings deposited in our lives' accounts needlessly.

Regarding Aloe, use it as a preventive measure; use it as a curative measure only as a last resort. This way, it will be much more lucrative for you. You will save money – because you will not need medicine. The universal need for dietary nutritional supplementation is no longer a question. It is essential to the preservation of good health and a long life.

Phenomena or reactions in your body

Using this Aloe, honey and distillate preparation either as preventive or as a curative measure may cause somewhat strange phenomena in your body. Don't worry. It is nature undertaking a purification process of the body through its excretion paths, a process that causes no harm to the body. Such phenomena are experienced when you use Aloe either as a preventive or as a curative measure.

It is important that you know how to recognize these phenomena when they happen.

Let's make some general observations about possible reactions that your body could manifest following the consumption of the Aloe preparation:

- The responses should not last a long time – a few hours, a few days, two or three at most.

- These reactions *must* occur! Their occurrence is proof that the detoxification and/or the healing from the illness is taking place.

- All the reactions are not experienced all at once. Normally, only one or two, rarely three, occur simultaneously.

- When these reactions surface, please do not become scared and suspend treatment. The presence of these phenomena are proof that healing is imminent; it is only a matter of time. You only need to continue the treatment to achieve definite healing. When you become aware of these phenomena, reduce the quantity to half the amount, since it is difficult to live with them. Once these reactions have disappeared, return with full confidence to the habitual dose.

- Your body will not be subjected to any type of harm. Rather, it will activate its release valves or, to put it another way, it will decide on its own to use its normal excretion paths and it will know which of them to use. It knows what's best for itself. Instead of being subjected to harm, it will go on to a progressive and total purification.

The body's excretion paths

The body has four means of excretion:

- The skin
- The feces
- The urine
- Vomiting

Normally, the body manifests two reactions:

- Pain
- Fever

The skin: If the body decides to purify itself through the skin, reactions you may experience range anywhere from a simple itch in the affected area, which could be anywhere on the body, all the way to an abscess, just to mention two extremes. Keep in mind that the itching sensation is not necessarily limited to only one spot of the body. In all likelihood, however, the actual response could be something that lies somewhere in the middle of these two extremes, such as some form of skin rash or blisters, namely rubella, measles, chicken pox or small-

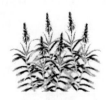

pox. If you develop a pimple or boil, do not think that you will go through the process of phlegmon or anthrax, things of the days of our grandparents.

To take care of the resulting condition, cut open an Aloe leaf and, leaving the skin on the outside, apply its internal part – the gel – on the area where the abscess has developed. Hold the Aloe leaf in place with a bandage. Whether you continue with the treatment is up to you. Immediately, you will experience a prickling of the skin, as if from a pin or bee sting. It is normal. It is Aloe expelling the impurities. You have done well. You are on the road to recovery.

The abscess will begin releasing all its contents within approximately three hours. Immediately see to the purification of the area. A lot of pus or bad blood or waste will come out. After cleaning the affected area, again apply the internal part of the leaf over the spot the pus has come out of. In the course of 24 hours, possibly less, you will notice that the infected area is painless and it has already healed. Fast healing? Too fast? It's because your blood is now a jewel. If the wound has difficulty closing over, it is because of the bad quality of the blood.

Feces: It is important to know that Aloe is a potent laxative. In fact, along with its worm property, traditional medicine makes wide use of this characteristic of Aloe. After a period of regular use of the preparation, you could notice a certain intestinal activity, including diarrhea, just to mention an extreme. It will regulate your intestine.

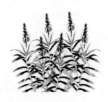

This phenomenon may last anywhere from a couple of hours up to three days at most. Nobody enjoys a laxative experience, even less so a very active person. You can decrease the quantity. If you were taking a full tablespoon's worth three times a day, cut it down to half the amount. In a short period of time, this symptom will disappear and everything will go back to normal. When everything is back to normal, slowly return to the normal dose.

Note: I repeat, Aloe has the ability to normalize your intestine.

Urine: Besides being a laxative, know that Aloe is also an excellent diuretic. After having used the preparation for some time, you could notice an increase in urination, with increased spontaneity and quantity. You could also notice that your urine may have a much more pronounced odor and color make-up. If the problem you wish to cure is linked to the liver (type A, B, C hepatitis or cirrhosis of the liver or a liver tumor – which, incidentally, Aloe has cured), the urine will be as dark as coffee or chocolate. This is because Aloe loosens up the gelatinous part of the liver, leaving behind a web-like tissue. Since the liver is the only organ of the body that reproduces itself, in a short period of time you will have a brand new liver. Proof can be found in the fact that before you started to take this preparation, any type of fried food or liquor gave you a great deal of discomfort, to say the least, but after taking our product, you

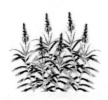

could have everything that a perfectly healthy person could have, without any consequences.

Vomiting: When we eat spoiled food, colonies of bacteria form and accumulate in the liver which, in an extreme struggle, tries to rid itself of these strange beings, inverting its peristaltic movements, and causing reflux. This phenomenon is known as vomiting, a major discomfort for all of us. Under the effect of Aloe, you may vomit, but it will be in the form of a single occurrence, without the typical antecedents of a sickness caused by spoiled food. Immediately after vomiting, our preparation will give you a feeling of relief, as if you had freed yourself of a burden.

In combination with the above-mentioned phenomena, you could also experience the following sensations:

Pain. Instantly, you may experience general aches and pains throughout the body, as if you have taken a long walk or have gone overboard with a sport or work activity that you are no longer used to doing. Where does this overall pain come from? It is the fact that you are now taking this product that has upset the "regularity" the body was used to. Nothing more.

If you are suffering from a localized problem, the pain may develop at that specific point. Let's give a practical example, for both a man as well as a woman:

- If you have a prostate problem, you may experience abdominal pain, a pain in the lower belly.

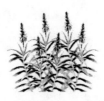

- A woman with a breast tumor may experience a pain in her armpit or in her ribcage or in her shoulder, somewhere in the general area of the affected breast.

Fever. In the evening, you may experience a barely perceptible fever without any apparent reason. It may be something like 99.5°F to 101.3°F. It will never be a high fever. There is no need to take any medication for it. It will go away all by itself.

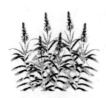

Part III

The Use of Aloe for the Cure of Illnesses

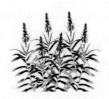

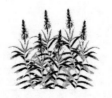

Introduction

We come across various lists of illnesses that suggest the possibility of using an Aloe-based treatment. The answers to some of the rare illnesses included in this list have been recently provided by science, whereas the more common ones have been inherited from past generations

In Cancer Can Be Cured!, in the chapter entitled *"Questions and Answers,"* two lists of illnesses are provided that can be cured with Aloe. In the treatment of illnesses, the first list generally makes use of the internal consumption of the Aloe, honey and distillate preparation. The second list, for the most part, deals with cases for which the topical application of the Aloe leaf is considered to be the best solution to the problem.

In that chapter, we record a list of the illnesses that are curable with Aloe, a list that we obtained from The Silent Healer, p. 40, by Bill Coats, R. Ph., and Robert Ahola. This list has been subsequently transcribed by Neil Stevens on page 65 of The Curative Power of Aloe (O poder curativo da babosa). In chapter 10 of this same book, on pages 101-104, we find "Uses of Aloe from A to Z." ("Usos da babosa de A a Z.")

In Part III of **Aloe Isn't Medicine, and Yet…It Cures!**, taking advantage of the list of illnesses from A to Z supplied by Neil Stevens, we would like to present, in the clearest and most concise way possible, the method by which to apply Aloe both internally and externally to treat and cure the illnesses. In his

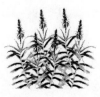

book, Stevens offers only an alphabetical listing of the illnesses that can be cured or treated with Aloe, without suggesting the application method. With the list in hand, then, let's explain how to use Aloe for the treatment of those illnesses.

Our job has been to take every illness in that list and find its definition. To this end, we have used **Dicionario Medico Andrei**, **Novo Dicionario Aurélio da Lingua Portuguesa** and the more contemporary **Dicionario Houaiss da Lingua Portuguesa.** These are the technical references used by the author for the original text in Portuguese whereas, for the purpose of this translation, the following reference texts have been used: **Il Gould Chiampo** (Zanichelli-McGraw-Hill, 1988) and **Webster's New Collegiate Dictionary,** (G. & C. Merriam Company, 1981).

We hope that with this information you will be able to solve the problems afflicting you at this time.

In line with this topic, Dr. Marie Lecardonnel, in **The New Guide to Aloe (O novo guia do Aloes – Receitas Praticas para sua saude),** Cascais/Portugal: Pubblicaçòes Prevençào da Saude, in Part III of her book of almost 300 pages, offers an exhaustive list of illnesses cured with Aloe, entitled: **Aloe and the Sickness from A to Z (De A a Z – O aloes e as doenças).**

Besides giving an alphabetical listing of the illnesses, Marie Lecardonnel's contribution to this topic includes the following:

- To give a technical description of how each disease is manifested;
- To give sensible advice to the patient;

- To provide the results of pertinent scientific studies on the subject;

- To recommend either the internal or external use of Aloe, as the case warrants; and

- To include testimonial accounts of healing by patients who have used Aloe as treatment.

In her book, Doctor Lecardonnel kindly mentions our recipe, directly or indirectly, almost one hundred times. She places us in Heaven on account of the "miraculous" results that people worldwide have obtained from using Aloe, for having dissemminated such a simple, economical, and effective recipe in a most rigorous Franciscan style, for the benefit of humanity, without a trace of discrimination, and for having encouraged everyone to make and use the home preparation.

In April of 2001, Vilson Francesco Bonacin sent us a floppy disk from Curitiba, PR, suggesting the title for the then proposed book. He suggested **Aloe Isn't Medicine, and Yet...It Cures! (Babosa nao é remédio, mas que cura, cura!)**. Besides suggesting the title, he also collaborated on the development of an alphabetical listing of the main illnesses, complete with a concise definition for each one of them. Bonacin selects 341 terms, many of which Neil Stevens had in his list. As you can see, this is more than double the number the American author used. In all honesty, the Paranean (he lived in Parana), in his eagerness to give hope and positive answers to the desperately ill, even includes some types of illnesses that positively cannot be cured with Aloe. For instance: caries, kleptomania, cross-eye, fracture, stammering, cleft lip, mongolism, etc. It would be dangerous to suggest or guarantee healing from these illnesses through the use of Aloe. For instance, the person who suffers from cross-eye would gain no improvement of his condition with Aloe. The person who suffers from caries would apply Aloe over the affected tooth but with no benefits. Whoever would use Aloe to treat kleptomania? It would be inconceivable to treat a broken thighbone with a topical application of Aloe without putting the leg in a cast! You don't correct a cleft lip with an Aloe potion. It would be unethical to mislead the people suffering from these diseases, knowing that the plant cannot and knows not how to help them. It would be panacea if it were so. However, the person who is suffering from the above diseases, or others, can take the Aloe, honey, and distillate preparation as a preventive measure, even though Aloe cannot resolve his problem. One needs to be honest.

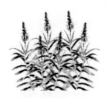

A

Abscess (anthrax, apostem, furuncle, phlegmon): A focus of suppuration (pus formation or discharge) within a tissue, organ, or region of the body.

Q. In the case of abscess caused by an accumulation of pus localized in different parts of the body, can I turn to Aloe?

A. Without a doubt.

Q. How?

A. By topical application.

Q. How do I proceed?

A. Imagine the plant's leaf. This leaf forms a complete unit as if it were two hands joined together. With a knife, open an Aloe leaf longitudinally (use one half as noted below and save the other half) and, without removing the skin, apply the internal part of the leaf – the gelatinous part – over the spot where the abscess has formed. Make sure the inside of the leaf is in direct contact with the inflamed area. Attach this piece of Aloe to an adhesive bandage and tap the area repeatedly. You will experience a pricking sensation as if by a needle. Congratulations on a job well done. It is the Aloe that is removing the pus from the ailing organic tissue. After a few hours, maybe three or four, it will explode. When you notice that it starts to ooze out, do a careful job of picking up that mixture of pus and bad blood. Once the medication is complete, use the other half of the leaf that you had put aside, repeating the treatment. Within 24 hours, the area will be regenerated, leaving it practically scar-free. Observe your skin. It's tender, red, healthy and free of the least bit of pain.

Remedy: Take the Aloe, honey and distillate preparation preemptively and avoid the inception of abscess. Taking this product is the same as purifying the blood. Abscesses are caused by the bad quality of the blood. If it is contaminated, the body collects the toxins and places them in the dustbin: the abscess. Blood is for the body what fuel is for the combustion engine. Ensuring optimal quality fuel guarantees long life for your car.

Acidity of the stomach (acid reflux, gastritis, gastric hyper-acidity, pyrosis) – Gastric hyperacidity: excessive concentration of acid, a painful burning sensation caused by gastroesophageal reflux (backflow from the stomach irritating the esophagus); symptomatic of an ulcer, a diaphragmatic hernia or other disorder. In these cases, can I use Aloe? If so, how?

Remedy: Make use of the Aloe recipe. A bottle will do it. In order to confirm it, take another one and eventually you can take a third bottle, without a long pause in between (three or four days, no more than a week). One option: have a piece of Aloe in your mouth during the day, swallowing the saliva.

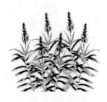

Another option: cut the Aloe leaf in very small parts, like you do with onions. Add water and then drink the water. Add more water when it is gone. After one or two hours, drink the water. Repeat it throughout the day

Acne: An inflammatory condition of the sebaceous glands common in adolescence and young adulthood, characterized by blackheads that often become inflamed and form papules, pustules, nodules, and cysts, usually on the face, chest, and back. **Juvenile acne:** Acne that is produced by hormonal changes, mainly by the androgenic and estrogenic types that normally occur in puberty.

Remedy: Rely on the home recipe of Aloe, honey and distillate. It will free the sebaceous glands. When acne manifests itself, apply small pieces of the Aloe leaf with their gel part right on the spot where the pimples show up, holding them in place with an adhesive bandage. Overnight, the Aloe will absorb the secretions and free the sebaceous glands without crushing or leaving a scar.

Addiction (on various drugs): Marked psychological and physiological dependence on a substance, such as alcohol or drugs, that has gone beyond voluntary control.

Remedy: Try the Aloe, honey and distillate preparation. Being a potent depurator (cleanser), Aloe has real potential to

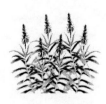

free the system of the toxins supplied by drugs. The same goes for the elimination of free radicals, a harmful substance in various pathological processes. By taking this product, you will notice a reduced yearning for alcohol, smoking, and drugs. Victory will be achieved with this reduction in yearning together with your will power.

AIDS: A condition of acquired immunological deficiency associated with infection of the cells of the immune system with the retrovirus HIV that occurs particularly in male homosexuals, drug addicts, and hemophiliacs. The major clinical forms of AIDS include opportunistic infections, Kaposi's sarcoma, other malignancies and lymphadenopathy (abnormal swelling of the lymph nodes). A very dangerous illness caused by a virus (HIV: *human immunodeficiency virus*, belonging to the group *retro-virus*) that destroys the immunological defenses of the body (*T lymphocytes*) and exposes the individual to various opportunistic infections: esophageal and bronchopulmonary candida, Cryptococcus disseminated in the central nervous system, interstitial pneumonia of the type *Pneumocysis carinii* or atypical microbacteria, toxoplasmosis, cytomycosis, herpes virus and cytomegalovirus infections and, at all stages of the illness, a few types of cancer (Kaposi's sarcoma, lymphoma). The blood tests may be positive (of the HIV carriers) for quite long periods of time (even for several years), before having clinical confirmation. The initial symptoms (pre-AIDS) consist of repeated bouts of fever, diarrhea, loss of weight, and lymphoadenopathy

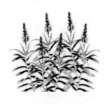

(enlarged lymph nodes glands). The first AIDS cases were discovered in the United States in 1979 in homosexuals, but it has been recorded that the illness also existed in various regions of equatorial Africa and in Haiti, again in homosexuals. Synonym: T epidemic immunity deficiency (CITE), acquired immune deficiency, acquired immunodeficiency syndrome, T epidemic immunodepression syndrome (SITE). World Health Organization (WHO) experts give the following definition of AIDS: the last stage is the most dangerous of a vast spectrum of pathologies associated with HIV.

Remedy: The use of the Aloe, honey and distillate preparation has cured AIDS. The therapy is long. Do not have prolonged intervals between jars, not more than three or four days, one week at the most. There is an abundance of literature that proves that Aloe cures AIDS. The explanation is simple: Aloe strengthens the immunological system, the weakest part of people suffering from AIDS. If the patient is taking a drug cocktail like AZT, he should also take Aloe. With time, he will be able to determine on his own that he can suspend the drug cocktail.

In 1985, Dr. Bill McAnalley isolated a polysaccharide taken from the Aloe vera, which he named "carrisyn." At the same time, Canadian researchers discovered an active molecule possessing remarkable antiviral properties, which they named "acemannan." Clinical tests on patients with AIDS showed that carrisyn could stop the pregression of the virus. This was

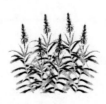

collaborated by the studies of several other researchers, notably by Dr. Reg McDaniel, who showed that, contrary to other treatments, the one based upon carrisyn showed no secondary effects. This was senstional news. Dr. McDaniel affirmed: "It seems that the carrisyn neutralizes the AIDS virus by transforming its protein envelope, thus preventing it from attacking the T4 cells. The preliminary report was published in 1987 in the Clinical Research Review: Aloe vera, the health and healing plant. **Note:** Carrisyn is the commercial name filed by the Carrington Laboratories for an Aloe-based medicine.

Allergies: A condition of acquired, specific alteration in biologic reactivity, initiated by exposure to an allergen and, after an incubation period, characterized by evocation of the altered reactivity upon re-exposure to the same or a closely related allergen. Hypersensitivity acquired by the body towards an extraneous substance (allergen), both of a normally inoffensive substance such as hair, dust, pollen, milk, etc., or of a medical or bacterial substance. It manifests an immediate reaction of different types: eczema, hives, spasmodic coryza, asthma.

Remedy: Because we are dealing with a weakened immune system, let's strengthen it with the preparation of Aloe, honey, and distillate. If necessary, repeat the treatment. If the allergy has produced inflammation or some type of harm to the skin, then we can turn to topical applications.

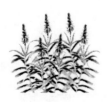

Alzheimer's Disease: Alzheimer's disease, which afflicts 24 million people worldwide, is the most common cause of dementia. Alzheimer's is a progressive and terminal disease for which there is no cure. In its most common form, it occurs in people over 65 years old. Supplements play a positive part in slowing the progress of some consequences of Alzheimer's.

Aloe is one of the most potent sources of antioxidants, including vitamins E and C and vitamin B-12 (only known natural source). Recent studies demonstrate the remarkable benefits of antioxidants. Oxidation in cells can damage DNA, leading sometimes to cancer, other diseases and to the changes associated with aging. The antioxidant compounds counter the aging effects wrought by free radicals.

Aloe vera has been shown to amplify the antioxidant effects of vitamins. It makes vitamin C, vitamin E and other anti-oxidants work better. It actually boosts the effects of antioxidants, probably due to its effect on enhancing blood quality and allowing the blood to more effectively transport oxygen and nutrients to the body's cells. Aloe vera makes everything nutritious work better due to its blood-enhancing effects. (See in bibliography: Vinson, J.A., Al Kharrat, H., Andreoli, L. Effect of Aloe vera preparations on the human bioavailability of vitamins C and E.)

Vitamin C (ascorbic acid) is a water-soluble vitamin essential to the prevention of scurvy. It is a commonly used supplement because there is epidemiological evidence that it reduces the risk of cancer, diabetes, cataracts, and Alzheimer's disease. This

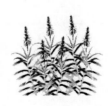

vitamin has been proven to increase absorption of iron and to improve poor iron status. A recent report showed that Aloe is unique in its ability to improve the absorption of both these vitamins and should be considered as an adjunct for people who take supplements.

Remedy: To the person who lives with this problem, I recommend taking the Aloe, honey, and distillate preparation. The fact that we do not have sound information that sheds light on this matter, either in theory or in practice, should not stop you from beginning to solve it. So make yourself the preparation. It will not hurt and will assist a person with Alzheimer's disease. Aloe has more than 300 useful substances, all important and essential for your body. It may be able to restore metabolism and glands to their normal function. It will also cleanse the body of toxins. Being intelligent, if the body thinks it needs something, it will search for it in its constant attempt to always perform at optimal efficiency.

Such a condition may be a sign of an overall deficiency in the body's immune system, so action must be taken to return it to good health. Let's try to purify the blood and its circulation. If the problem is something else, the Aloe, honey, and distillate preparation will help the body find a solution to the problem.

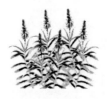

Plan on taking the Aloe, honey, and distillate preparation for a period of anywhere from three to six months continuously (if you take a break between jars, make sure it isn't longer than three or four days, a week at the very most). Such therapy helps restore the body's normal activities. It also serves as a defense against the disease.

See McDaniel, H. Reg., M.D.: Response of Alzheimer's Disease to extended micronutrition in Bibliography.

Anemia: A reduction below normal in erythrocytes, hemoglobin, or hematocrit. A hemoglobin and/or erythrocyte deficiency in the blood. One speaks of anemia when the hemoglobin concentration is below 13 grams per 100ml for men and 11 grams per 100ml for women. Anemia manifests itself through various symptoms: paleness of the skin and of the mucosa, vertigo (dizziness), tachycardia, and digestive ailments

Remedy: An anemic person manifests some weaknesses. In this condition, the person ought to take a series of successive jars of the Aloe, honey and distillate preparation.

Note: In the case of pure and simple anemia, topical application of Aloe is not deemed appropriate.

Anorexia: Absence of appetite. A syndrome of unknown cause characterized by profound aversion to food, leading to emaciation and sometimes serious nutritional deficiencies; usually seen in young women.

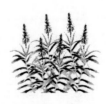

Remedy: To correct this dysfunction, it is sufficient to take the Aloe, honey and distillate preparation. However, if the anorexia is of a mental or nervous origin, the patient should consult a psychologist so the origin of the condition may be identified. I would like to caution mainly the western female part of society to beware of drugs that promise fast weight loss. Besides making your wallets lighter, they can harm your health!

Anthrax: An acute infectious disease of cattle and sheep, transmissible to man and caused by *Bacillus anthracis*. A carbuncle or malignant pustule.

Remedy: Because we are dealing with an infection, take the Aloe, honey and distillate preparation. It may yield excellent results.

Aphonia: Loss of speech due to peripheral lesions, as in laryngeal paralysis or vocal cord tumor.

Remedy: Use only the home recipe of Aloe, honey and distillate. If the problem persists after the first jar, repeat until the problem is solved. However, if the symptoms persist after three or four jars worth of treatment, consult a doctor.
Note: In such case, the external or topical use of the leaf does not seem to be appropriate.

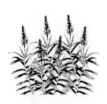

Aphtha or ulcer: A white painful oral ulcer of unknown cause.

Remedy: The Aloe, honey and distillate preparation will slowly take care of the problem. When the body has been decongested, it will free itself of various types of problems.

Regarding oral and genital aphtha, the problem is easily resolved with topical applications. Apply small pieces of the leaf (the gelatinous part) right on the affected area. If you do this application before going to sleep, the condition will be corrected by morning. Try it, and you will be able to confirm this. Topical application is a first aid remedy.

If the patient is a newborn, two or three drops of the Aloe, honey, and distillate preparation is an adequate treatment. A couple of days later, increase the quantity to a teaspoonful.

Heart and Kidney

- **Arterial failure:** Inability of an organ to fully perform its normal functions.
- **Aortic regurgitation:** Backflow of blood from the aorta into the left ventricle through or around an abnormal or prosthetic aortic valve.
- **Heart failure:** The condition in which the heart is no longer able to pump an adequate supply of blood in relation to venous return and to meet the metabolic needs of body tissues.

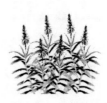

- **Coronary insufficiency:** Prolonged precordial pain or discomfort without conventional evidence of myocardial infarction; subendocardial ischemia due to a disparity between coronary blood flow and myocardial needs.
- **Mitral regurgitation:** Imperfect closure of the mitral valve during the cardiac systole, permitting blood to re-enter the left atrium.
- **Renal failure:** A reduction in kidney function, acute or chronic, to a level at which the kidneys are unable to maintain normal biological homeostasis.
- **Acute renal insufficiency:** Rapid decline in renal function followed by physiological and biochemical abnormalities, as in acute tubular necrosis; generally due to damage of renal parenchyma by intrinsic disease or extrinsic factors.
- **Respiratory insufficiency:** Incompetence of the respiratory processes.
- **Tricuspid regurgitation:** Reflux of blood into the right atrium during ventricular systole, due to incomplete or inadequate closure of the tricuspid valve.

Remedy: Why has this organ (heart or kidney) lost its ability to carry out its functions? Let's try to restore this ability by getting the Aloe, honey and distillate preparation ready.

Arteriosclerosis: Any of various proliferative and degenerative changes in arteries, not necessarily related to each other, resulting in thickening of the walls, loss of elasticity, and in

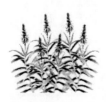

some instances, calcium deposition. A degenerative disease of the arteries caused by the destruction of the smooth muscular fibers and of the elastic fibers that it is made up of, causing the hardening of arterial walls. It is generally caused by long lasting arterial hypertension or by aging.

Remedy: The solution is to take the Aloe, honey and distillate preparation frequently. The healing process may take anywhere from three to six months. If you take a break between jars, make sure it is brief.

Arthritis: Inflammation of a joint. It can be acute or chronic, as a result of a trauma or an illness (acute articular rheumatism, gout, evolutionary/developmental chronic polyarthritis, blennorrhea, etc.).

Remedy: Take a successive series of jars of the Aloe, honey and distillate preparation. The topical application will give relief from the pain in the inflamed joints. The therapy is slow, but it may resolve the problem.

Note: If the patient makes use of our preparation, with time he can do without the topical applications, which he can always turn back to at any time.

Asthma: A disease characterized by an increased responsiveness of the trachea and bronchi to various stimuli (often allergens) and manifested by widespread airway narrowing

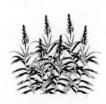

that changes in severity either spontaneously or as a result of therapy; present as episodic dyspnea (difficult or labored respiration), cough, and wheezing.

Remedy: A successive series of jars of the Aloe, honey and distillate preparation will free the bronchi of extraneous matter accumulated there, allowing the diaphragm to resume its normal functioning.

Athlete's foot (Tinea Pedis): Fungus infection of the feet, especially the webs of the toes and the soles. Caused by Epidermophyton flocculosum, various species of Tricophyton, and rarely by Microsporum.

Remedy: For this condition, we recommend the topical application, the direct contact of the gelatinous part of the Aloe leaf with the affected area. Perform this operation for the entire day, repeating it three or four times in a 24-hour period. It is also advised that after every washing up, the person who suffers from this ailment dry very well the area between the toes with antiseptic talc. In addition, we propose an occasional jar of Aloe, honey, and distillate preparation; it will certainly not cause any harm.

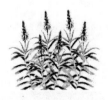

B

Baldness: Absence of hair. Definitive loss of hair, total or partial; this is frequently caused by seborrhea of the scalp and it affects almost exclusively men.

Remedy: Ancient people, including our American Mayas, knew of and used Aloe as a hair tonic. The use of Aloe rejuvenates and strengthens hair, giving it more shine and its natural color. Using the Aloe, honey and distillate preparation will fight the causes of baldness, ensuring that the body regains what it lost along the way, mainly due to a bad diet.

Note: Besides taking Aloe internally, apply it on the scalp, combined with gentle massages. The massages will aid the blood circulation in the affected area which, if the roots are not dead, may lead to a reactivation of hair growth. So do not be surprised if, slowly, your desert turns into forest again. You will not be the first person to experience this phenomenon.

Birthmarks *(skin spots, age spots):* Change in the coloration of the skin without either elevation or depression.

Remedy: Research done by Dr. Ivan E. Danhof has revealed that "Aloe penetrates into the skin at least four times as fast as water." Such capability is the benefit of lignin, a substance that aids penetration into the skin. The resulting benefit of this is that the affected area is supplied with all the substances it needs very quickly. In addition, as a pleasant, unexpected consequence, you will also get soft, hydrated, rejuvenated, tender, and lubricated skin. As a practical application, use the Aloe, honey and distillate preparation. This preparation creates a favorable environment for the development of healthy skin.

In relation to birthmarks and other general skin spots, to speed up the clearing process, in addition to using the preparation, apply the plant's juice topically on the spot you wish to eliminate. This will yield faster results.

Blisters: A vesicle (cyst) resulting from the exudation of serous fluid between the epidermis and dermis.

Remedy: Topical application only. Open up an Aloe leaf. Apply its gelatinous interior on the spot where the blister is, holding it in place with an adhesive bandage. Aloe will see to it that the serosity, the lymph, the pus or the blood that is collected under the skin is expelled.

Bronchitis: Inflammation of the mucous membrane of the bronchi.

Remedy: Bcause we are dealing with inflammation, our preparation of Aloe, honey and distillate can be the answer. If one jar's worth does not yield the desired results, take as much as necessary to achieve your goal.

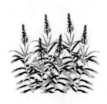

Bruises: An injury producing capillary hemorrhage below an unbroken skin. Harm done by a blow or impact, without causing the laceration or rupture of the skin; trauma.

Remedy: A bruise is caused by a blow or an impact to an area of healthy tissues. At times it causes a hematoma – the formation of blood in the tissue – as a result of the trauma and as a consequence of the rupturing of blood vessels. Quickly turn to the Aloe leaf. You may crush it, you may grind it in a blender, or simply open it up with a knife and then apply it over the affected area. Being analgesic, Aloe will have the immediate effect of alleviating the pain. If you keep it on the affected area for a period of at least 24 hours, it will reduce the hematoma and even eliminate it. Taking the Aloe, honey and distillate preparation may speed up your recovery process.

Burns (thermal, radiation, solar, chemical or liquid types): The tissue reaction or injury resulting from application of heat, extreme cold, caustics, radiation, friction, or electricity; classified as simple hyperemic (first degree), vesicant (second degree), destructive of skin and underlying tissues (third degree). We recognize four different burn levels: **first degree burns,** with painful redness and swelling; **second degree burns,** with the presence of blisters; **third degree burns**, a case where the blisters become worse due to the necrosis of the derma and, at times, of the sub-adjacent parts; **fourth degree burns,** carbonization of an entire area of the body.

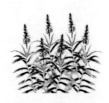

Remedy: Immediately apply Aloe topically. Cut the leaf open, apply the gel part of the leaf over the wound, holding it in place with a bandage (adhesive or cloth type) regardless of the degree of burn. You will experience an almost immediate relief from the pain. With the exception of the case where the burned area is reduced to carbon (a phase beyond the third degree burns of the above definition), expect a total and very fast recovery. Taking an eventual jar of the Aloe, honey and distillate preparation as a supplement will serve to speed up the recovery.

Bursitis: Inflammation of a bursa.

Remedy: Because we are dealing with an inflammatory process, the Aloe, honey and distillate preparation is like manna from the sky. The treatment will be a bit slow but, with perseverance, you will achieve your objective of alleviating the pain without resorting to injections that help to calcify the area. Remember that Aloe works quietly and lubricates. Do not be afraid to repeat the treatment. Repeat it as many times as is necessary to solve your problem.

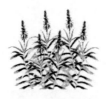

C

Cancer: A malignant tumor. Any disease characterized by malignant tumor formation or proliferation of anaplastic cells. The uncontrollable and incessant proliferation of any anarchical (out of control) cell that generally invades the tissues and has the ability to metastasize in various parts of the body and is potentially recidivous, even after surgical interventions; it can cause death if not properly cured; malignant tumor (generally, this term is used when referring to carcinoma).

Remedy: There are hundreds of different types of cancer, ranging from very aggressive ones to slow ones that an individual can live with for a prolonged period of time, and benign ones. With any type of cancer, it doesn't matter which organ is affected. Immediately begin taking the Aloe, honey and distillate preparation. Cures have been recorded of all types of cancer. Today, after 20 years of use, day after day, thousands of people in the entire world are cured of this disease. The human body heals itself and nutrition derived from the Aloe arborescens plant provides the resources to accomplish the work.

In 2002, according to the Padua, Italy experiment of three years of work, under the attention of a scientific group coordinated by the director of the Institute of Microbiology at the University of Padua, Professor Giorgio Palu, Professor Modesto Carli (oncologist and pediatrician) and Doctor Teresa

Pecere, who has a degree in natural science and is a researcher in molecular biology, Aloe has the ability to reverse the proliferation of the anaplastic cells. (See bibliography Pecere, T., Carli, M., Palu, G.)

Here's the miracle! Hence, the cells, reconstituted in health instead of producing carcinogenic (sick) cells, will generate healthy cells. In other words, you have been cured of your cancer. For more complete details on how this recipe has helped people in their cancer fight read **Cancer Can Be Cured!**, the first book by Father Romano Zago.

But it isn't enough to take the Aloe, honey and distillate preparation as if it were a magic wand that will make this disease disappear magically. There is no such magic wand! There is no such magic! You must convert yourself. You must recognize your mistakes, your excesses, and alter your way of life and your diet. You must make adjustments in every sense: physical, psychic, emotional, spiritual. You must be willing to give up that former, improper lifestyle and adopt other forms, more positive ones, more constructive ones, and live this new discovery with gusto as if to make up for lost time and ground. And you will succeed! You have discovered a new, better reality, and you want to live life, the greatest gift of this world, more intensely and in good health.

Have regular clinical check-ups. Preferably, have them with the doctor who diagnosed your illness. The result of such analysis will convince you to continue with the treatment, either by increasing the dose or by taking breaks.

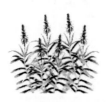

Candidiasis: A condition produced by infection with a fungus of the genus Candida, usually *C. albicans;* involving various parts of the body, such as skin, mucous membrane, nails, bronchi, lungs, heart, vagina, and gastrointestinal tract, and rarely, the occurrence of septicemia. Intense, subacute or chronic affliction, caused by excrescences pertinent to the genus Candida (mostly **Candida albicans**). The infection affects mainly the skin and the mucosa, and it manifests itself in the form of rashes of small white pustules. Infection due to fungi of the species *Candida* or *Monilia albicans*, which generally infect the labial commessura, the mouth, the oropharynx, the vagina and the gastrointestinal tract; moniliasis.

Remedy: We are happy to inform our readers that the Aloe, honey and distillate preparation cures candidiasis. If you have such a problem, turn to this preparation.

Cataract: Partial or complete opacity of the crystalline lens or its capsule.

Remedy: Let me explain better. A cataract is a kind of veil that, with time, forms in the crystalline lens, a transparent lenticular body located in the front part of the vitreous humor of the eye. Medical practice is to remove the crystalline lens. If you are patient, you may be able to avoid surgery. All you need do is apply one drop of the juice of an Aloe leaf into the affected eye. If you experience any type of inflammation, you will feel it

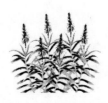

burn. If this burning sensation is terribly strong, practically intolerable, dilute that natural juice with a physiological solution, in a one-to-one ratio, more or less. You will notice a decrease in the discomfort.

Applying this solution various times a day will be like slowly scratching that veil until, with time, it will be completely destroyed, restoring the crystalline lens to its natural transparency.

If you wish to speed up this process, it can be done very simply. About half an hour, more or less, after applying the Aloe juice into the eye, apply a small drop of honey in the eye. Reacting to this external substance, the eyelid will become more active, thus collaborating to wear away the tissue of that veil. At this point, it would be ideal if the patient went to an ophthalmologist, an expert in the field, who would proceed to remove the remains of the veil.

Catarrh: Inflammation of mucous membranes, especially those of the air passages, associated with mucoid exudate. Catarrh is an old term that designates an intense or chronic inflammation of the mucosa; presently reserved exclusively for the inflammation of the respiratory tracts accompanied by abundant secretions. In everyday language, saliva or mucus, at times mixed with pus or blood, originating in the mucosa of the respiratory tracts: oropharynx, trachea, bronchi, and expelled through the mouth.

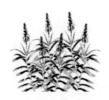

Remedy: Prepare the Aloe, honey and distillate preparation. One jar should be enough, but if there is need for a second, do not be stingy.

Cellulitis: A diffuse inflammation of connective tissue, especially of subcutaneous tissue, manifesting itself in the form of a hardened mass, at times painful, affecting mainly women's thighs and buttocks.

Remedy: We have already repeated that, when dealing with inflammation, the Aloe, honey and distillate preparation is effective. Besides taking the oral preparation, follow the advice of the experts with exercises, massages, walks, etc. The vanity of keeping a young and toned body motivates millions, but with modest returns. It is unlikely that never before in the course of history has mankind spent so much money on the care of the body in the attempt to keep it young and beautiful. *"Vanitas vanitatum!"*

Cirrhosis: 1 Hepatic cirrhosis: Any diffuse fibrosis that destroys the normal lobular architecture of the liver with destruction and regeneration of hepatic parenchymal cells. **2 Interstitial inflammation:** Interstitial inflammation of any tissue or organ. A chronic and serious illness of the liver where the normal parenchyma (functional elements of the organ) undergoes an extensive and progressive fibrous transformation. A cirrhotic liver appears pinkish, hard and bumpy. Cirrhosis is caused by a

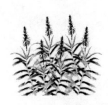

number of things: alcoholism, a bad diet, viral hepatitis complications, etc.

Remedy: Because Aloe is bitter, the liver accepts it readily. Therefore, take the Aloe, honey and distillate preparation. We have recorded cases of complete healing from hepatic cirrhosis types A, B and C as well as from liver tumors. Aloe restores the liver integrally. However, it is stressed that the patient modify his eating and drinking habits.

Cold: A mild, acute, contagious, upper respiratory viral infection of short duration, characterized by coryza, watering of the eye, cough, and occasionally, fever.

Remedy: Only a weakened immune system catches a cold. If the body's defenses were intact, even in the event of direct contact, the virus would not be allowed to develop. Therefore, practice prevention! Take the Aloe, honey, and distillate preparation regularly as a preventive measure. It will prevent colds. However, even if you have already contracted the virus, once you experience its debilitating effects, with shivers, congestion of the respiratory tracts, headaches, inflammation of the throat, etc., do not hesitate: prepare the Aloe, honey, and distillate preparation. Taking it will aid the body's defenses to fight the invader and speed up the healing process.

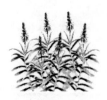

Colic: Acute paroxysmal abdominal pain usually due to smooth muscle contraction, obstruction, or twisting.

Remedy: The main and the best known ones are biliary colic, hepatic colic, gastric colic, intestinal colic, menstrual colic, and kidney colic. If you have these problems, turn to the Aloe, honey and distillate preparation. Aloe decongests the obstructed organ. The obstruction is generally caused by bad digestion or imbalanced diet. Our preparation has even been successful in removing stones formed in the kidneys and in the gall bladder.

Colitis: Inflammation of the colon, total or of a segment, of an infectious origin (bacterial or amebic), caused by the bad digestion of some food or by an unbalanced diet, or by unknown causes, such as ulcerative colitis, commonly called ulcerous-hemorrhagic.

Remedy: Once you have determined your condition, rely on the Aloe, honey and distillate preparation to resolve your problem. There is no need to take a large number of jars. However, it would be wise on your part to take a few jars a year of the Aloe preparation for optimal system fitness. At what intervals? You decide. Just to refresh your memory, read again Part II, chapter 5 – *"Aloe as preventive measure."*

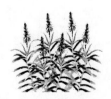

Congestion: An abnormal accumulation of fluid within the vessels of an organ or part; usually blood, but occasionally bile or mucus.

Remedy: There are several types of congestions. There is intestinal congestion, nasal congestion, cerebral congestion, venous congestion, pleuropulmonary congestion, kidney congestion, facial congestion, mucous congestion, congestion of the bile, etc. As the names imply, congestion is the accumulation of an extraneous body in an organ. The Aloe, honey and distillate preparation will act to unblock this obstructed area by removing the abnormalities that contributed to the development of this condition.

Cough: The act of expelling air suddenly and violently from the lungs after deep inspiration and closure of the glottis; a protective reflex caused by irritation of the laryngeal, tracheal, or bronchial mucosa.

Remedy: We have various types of coughs: long cough, whooping cough, convulsive cough, canine cough, and dry cough that does not lead to expectoration.

It is clear that you cannot afford to come down with any type of cough. If you commit to taking the Aloe, honey, and distillate preparation regularly, you can avoid these setbacks. Likewise, take the Aloe preparation even when you come down with a cough. Continue this therapy until you are free of this

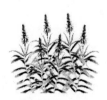

discomfort. As you know, in matters of health, prevention is the best cure.

Cuts: An opening made with an edged or sharp instrument.

Remedy: In the case of accidents of this nature, turn to an open Aloe leaf. You don't happen to have a bottle of hydrogen peroxide available to disinfect the cut? Don't worry. Aloe, which is also a disinfectant, will provide this service as well, and gratuitously. Applying the gelatinous, inner part of the Aloe leaf over the affected area disinfects the wound. If the wound is bleeding, you will notice that, besides giving you relief from the pain, it will also stop the bleeding in two minutes. Held in place, the piece of leaf will heal the cut in one or two days. If the cut is so large as to require stitching, then the Aloe leaf can be applied over the stitches, speeding up considerably the healing process and reducing scarring.

Cystitis: Inflammation of the urinary bladder. Acute or chronic inflammation of the mucosa of the bladder, generally of an infectious source.

Remedy: When dealing with inflammation, turn to the benefits of the Aloe, honey and distillate preparation. The results are fast in coming.

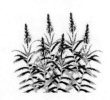

D

Dandruff: Scales of greasy keratotic material shed from the scalp.

Remedy: Aloe does an excellent job of fighting dandruff. It is sufficient to turn to topical applications. Therefore, grind Aloe leaves and apply the pulp-like substance over the scalp, massaging the area. Such treatment must be repeated indefinitely. However, why not attack the problem at the root? How? Prepare the Aloe, honey and distillate preparation and take it orally. Only a system in precarious health, with frequent colds, sore throat, and catarrh, develops dandruff. As the Aloe plant offers more than 300 useful substances, all important and essential for the body, these substances are able to replenish the body with the ingredients it lacks, bringing back good health and eliminating the source of this condition. In short: together with the topical application, turn to the benefits that the Aloe, honey and distillate preparation has to offer.

Depression: A state of feeling sad. A psycho-neurotic or psychotic disorder marked by sadness, inactivity, difficulty in thinking and concentration, and feelings of dejection. A state of discouragement, loss of interest arising from losses, disappointments, physical and psychic stress, when the individual becomes aware of his suffering and of the sense of isolation that surrounds him. The psychic aspect perseveres for long periods and recurrent depressive dysphoria, coinciding with real or imaginary problems or with momentary experiences of suffering, and could be accompanied by perturbation of the mind.

Remedy: Depression is always linked with the immune system. When this system is weak, on account of a decrease in blood pressure and in body temperature, we can come down with the above-mentioned symptoms. Get the Aloe, honey and distillate preparation ready at once. Thanks to the innumerable medicinal properties contained in the Aloe plant, within little time you will successfully come out of that depressing state.

Dermatitis: An inflammation of the skin. Any type of inflammation of the skin; dermatitis. Atypical dermatitis, the same as eczema (acute or chronic allergic infection of the skin), that shows up as an inflammatory reaction with the formation of blisters, the development of scales and itching. **Contact dermatitis:** caused by the contact of the skin with a specific allergen, such as resin, cosmetics, some vegetables, etc., marked by erythema, edema and the presence of blisters in the exposed spot. **Dermatitis seborrheica:** produces macular and scariforme rashes that show up mainly on the face, on the scalp, in the chest and in the pubic area.

Remedy: The various types of dermatitis manifestations, explained above, deal with the inflammation caused by both

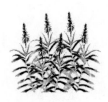

major and minor infections. The appropriate prescription is Aloe, honey and distillate. There is a good chance of success, even more so if we are dealing with the more serious cases such as seborrheic dermatitis. Combine the oral preparation with the topical application of the Aloe leaf.

Diabetes: A disease characterized by the habitual discharge of an excessive quantity of urine and by excessive thirst.

Remedy: American literature assures us that Aloe cures diabetes. Twenty years of practice in direct daily contact with this plant and the patients who have used it confirm this statement. We have documented the cure of diabetics who had used insulin for twenty years. Using our preparation, they have been able to bring their blood values within the normal limits in a matter of six months, allowing them to do away with the insulin injection. Therefore, we recommend the Aloe, honey and distillate preparation as a cure for diabetes. Relative to honey and diabetes, please see part I, chap. 5 – *"Honey in the case of diabetes."*

Dislocations: The displacement of one or more bones of a joint or of any organ from the original position.

Remedy: Twisting, sprains, stretching, dislocations, all call for topical applications. Aloe-based remedies do exist, but they are expensive. In their place, you can grind an entire leaf and

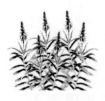

apply the resultant product over the traumatized area. Because of its great penetration capability, you will experience almost immediate relief from the pain. If the bone or the nerve has really been dislocated, seek the services of a traumatologist to set it back in position.

Ever since the 1976 Olympic Games in Montreal, Canada, we have received reports of athletes who have turned to the Aloe gel, together with aspirin, to obtain relief from the pain caused by sprains and swelling. We learn from others' experiences. How pleasant it is to know that there are people who share their positive experiences with the community!

Discouragement: Deprivation of confidence

Remedy: We are dealing with a slow process of depersonalization, which can lead to more serious psychological dysfunctions potentially capable of leading the individual to commit such extreme acts as suicide. The psychological state of discouragement defined above is an indication of the weakened state of the immune system. Here we have proof that the human being is one entity. Discouragement seems to be located in the psychological area of a person, even though its cause can be found in the physical side.

The Aloe, honey, and distillate preparation works well for psychological illnesses. Your aim is to strengthen the immune system. The preparation will give you a welcome push.

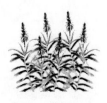

Distension: Distension or dislocation of a tissue or of an organ (muscles, ligaments, nerves, etc.). **Abdominal distension:** an increase of the abdominal volume due to a physiological condition (for example, pregnancy) or pathological (for example, ascites, intestinal obstruction, tumor, etc.). **Muscular distension:** breakage of a muscle's ligaments due to excessive violent traction; muscular stretching.

Remedy: For relief from abdominal distension, take the Aloe, honey and distillate preparation. In the case of a muscular distension, turn to the topical application of the Aloe leaf after grinding it to a pulp. Apply the pulp over the traumatized area and hold it in place with a bandage. Keep it there overnight; it will speed up the healing process. You can also seek the services of a professional masseur.

Dysentery: Inflammation of the intestine, particularly the colon, from various causes associated with abdominal pain, tenesmus (inability to have a bowel movement), and diarrhea with blood and mucus.

Remedy: Aloe is a potent bactericide. If the dysentery is caused by bacteria, the Aloe, honey and distillate preparation gives a realistic possibility of success.
Note: The fact that Aloe is a laxative as well does not mean that this preparation would harm the patient. The use of Aloe

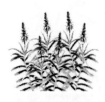

regulates the intestine, both the naturally lazy intestine as well as the one affected with dysentery.

E

Edema: Excessive accumulation of fluid in the tissue spaces due to increased transudation of the fluid from the capillaries. **Pulmonary edema:** An effusion of fluid into the air sacs and interstitial tissue of the lungs, producing severe dyspnea; most commonly due to left heart failure. **Angioedema:** An acute, transitory, localized, painless swelling of the subcutaneous tissue or submucosa of the face, hands, feet, genitalia, or viscera. It may be hereditary or caused by a food or drug allergy, an infection, or by emotional stress.

Remedy: Whatever your type of edema, being that we are dealing with an accumulation of liquids or with an inflammation, infection or trauma, turn to the Aloe, honey and distillate preparation. There are possibilities for recovery. You can't make it worse.

Enteritis: Any inflammation of the intestinal tract, especially of the mucosa.

Remedy: Because we are dealing with inflammation, let the Aloe, honey and distillate preparation take care of this.

Remember that Aloe is a powerful laxative; in the end it will regulate your intestine. This is a great benefit!

Epidermitis: Inflammation of the outer layer of the skin.

Remedy: Once again we are dealing with an inflammation, so the answer lies in the Aloe, honey, and distillate preparation. It likes to make itself useful this way. Give it a try.

Epstein-Barr virus: Herpes-like virus particles first noted in cultured human lymphoblasts from Burkitt's malignant lymphoma, and of uncertain significance as etiologic agents of such tumors. These viruses may be the cause of, or related to, infectious mononucleosis .

Remedy: Infection. Lymphoma. Cancer. We offer the Aloe, honey, and distillate preparation to fight the illness.

Eruption/Rash: Eruption: The sudden appearance of lesions on the skin, especially in exanthematous diseases and sometimes as a result of a drug. **Rash:** A lay term used for nearly any skin eruption but more commonly for acute inflammatory dermatosis.

Remedy: The definition refers to "lesions of an inflammatory or infective nature." The Aloe, honey and distillate preparation fights inflammation and infection. To aid the healing process,

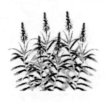

you can use the topical application of the Aloe leaf over the area where the rash has developed.

Erysipelas: A form of acute streptococcal cellulitis involving the skin, with a well-demarcated, slightly raised red area having advancing borders, usually accompanied by constitutional symptoms.

Remedy: We are dealing with an infection, so let the Aloe, honey and distillate preparation disinfect the system. It will not harm the healing process. To speed it up even more, we recommend a topical application over the area with these red spots.

Exanthema: An eruption on the skin. Any eruptive fever or disease.

Remedy: Disinfecting an ailing system is the Aloe, honey and distillate preparation's trademark contribution. It will surely give excellent results in the case of exanthema (rashes) as well.

Eye diseases: Biological alteration of the state of health of a being (human or animal) that manifests through a multitude of symptoms, perceptible or non; infirmity, illness, pain (cancer is an illness that is very difficult to cure). See **Myopia** and **Presbyopia** in this alphabetical listing.

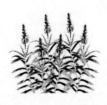

Remedy: Any type of eye infection can be cured with the juice from the Aloe leaf. Take advantage of the disinfecting power of Aloe.

Other preventable illnesses

Remedy: Take a jar of Aloe, honey, and distillate preparation. This treatment will prevent these illnesses:
- Headaches – internal use;
- Tooth aches – topical application;
- Stomach aches – internal use;
- Muscular aches – massage;
- Articulation (joint) pains – massage;

The key for each type of pain is to know its origin.
- Why have you got a headache?
- Why have you got a tooth ache?
- Why have you got a stomach ache?
- Why have you got muscle aches?
- Why have you got articulation (joint) pains?

We have known for a long time that Aloe is an analgesic. Therefore, whenever you have any kind of body pain and its source is from within, turn to the Aloe, honey, and distillate preparation, which never hurts. On the other hand, if the pain is the result of a blow by a blunt object, turn to the topical application of the Aloe leaf. Applying a piece of leaf over the traumatized area will, at minimum, alleviate the pain. Take tooth aches, for instance. If the cause is cavities, it is obvious you need a filling; Aloe can only alleviate the pain. Cavities must be treated by a specialist. Had there been a preventive therapy in effect, who knows if cavities would have developed in the first place? Aloe is rich in calcium. Now that you have spotted cavities, place yourself under the expert care of your dentist. It's the only way to treat this problem.

F

Fever (for no apparent reason): Elevation of the body temperature above the normal; in human beings, above an average value of 98.6°F (37°C) orally.

Remedy: The increase in body temperature signals the presence of foreign matter in the body. It is not sufficient to turn to an antithermic, effective only in lowering the temperature. It is important to search for the causes of such rise in temperature. In short: why do I have a fever? Where did it come from? Regardless of the type of fever, the Aloe, honey and distillate preparation can lower the temperature to its normal value.

Fissures: Any groove or cleft normally occurring in a part or organ such as the skull, liver, or spinal cord. A crack in skin or an ulcer in mucous membrane. Small longitudinal fissure, wound, rupture, groove, any deep or superficial ulceration. A wound in the callous skin of the hands or of the feet, generally of people who perform heavy, physical work.

Remedy: This problem is similar in nature to all the other skin problems we have seen so far. Therefore, we repeat the same wise suggestions we have expressed for those cases – topical application, meaning placing the gelatinous part of the leaf over the affected area. Other sound advice would be to turn to the Aloe, honey and distillate preparation because the cause of the injury is a lack of lubrication. Likewise for the lips. Know that Aloe contains lubricating fluids.

Flatulence: The presence or sensation of excessive gas in the stomach and intestinal tract.

Remedy: This condition can be eliminated only with the use of the Aloe, honey and distillate preparation taken orally. The origin of such turbulence probably lies with an inappropriate diet for the liver and the stomach.

Fungus: A low form of plant life, a division of the thallophytes without chlorophyll. The chief classes of fungi are the phycomycetes, Ascomycetes, Basidiomycetes, and Fungi Imperfecti. Most of the pathogenic fungi belong to the last group. A spongy morbid excrescence. **The Novo Dicionàrio Larousse Cultural**

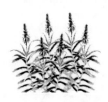

da Lìngua Portuguesa says about it: "fleshy, spongy excrescence that appears on the skin, especially around a wound and that has the appearance of a mushroom."

Remedy: People can tackle this problem with topical applications of Aloe, since the plant is a fungicide. Taking the Aloe, honey and distillate preparation orally can help remove the parasite, eliminating the problem at the root. The treatment may be slow in giving results, but it works.

Furuncle (Boil pimple): A localized infection, usually staphylococcal, of skin and subcutaneous tissue, which usually originates in or about a hair follicle and develops into a solitary abscess that drains externally through a single suppurating tract; a boil.

Remedy: Follow the same procedure recommended for abscess, since they are the same.

G

Gangrene: 1. Necrosis of a part; due to failure of the blood supply, to disease, or to direct injury. 2. The putrefactive changes in dead tissue.

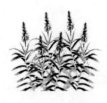

Remedy: Make the topical application treatment, but also take the oral preparation of Aloe, honey and distillate. The necrosis will be cleared up after some time.

Gingivitis: Inflammation of the gingiva, the mucous membrane and underlying soft tissue that covers the alveolar process and surrounds a tooth.

Remedy: Group under the title "gum inflammation" or "gum diseases," all the pathological or infectious conditions of the mouth: gums fistula, inflammation of the mucosa, and even dental surgery and/or tooth extraction. If you develop such problems, turn to topical application of the Aloe leaf. Cut it open and apply its gelatinous part over the affected area. Keep it on overnight.

Infections of this nature find their origin in metabolism. An occasional preparation of Aloe, honey and distillate will help to avoid these setbacks: *prevention is the best cure!*, as the saying wisely has it.

Glaucoma: An eye disease, the complete clinical picture of which is characterized by increased intraocular pressure, excavation and degeneration of the optic nerve head, and typical nerve fiber bundle defects that produce characteristic defects in the visual field. May be primary, secondary, or congenital.

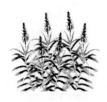

Remedy: Such a condition is a sign of an overall deficiency in the body's immune system, so action must be taken to return it to good health. The considerable resources present in the Aloe, honey and distillate preparation are exactly what you need to do just that.

Gout: 1. Primary gout, an inborn error of uric acid metabolism characterized by hyperuricemia and recurrent attacks of acute arthritis, most often of the great toe, and eventually by tophaceous deposits of urates; 2. Secondary gout, the gouty symptom complex, which may be acquired as a complication of polycythemia vera and other myeloproliferative disorders, as well as of diuretic therapy.

Remedy: In essence, the patient has an excess of uric acid in the body. Let's go and destroy this accumulation. In the meantime, use the Aloe, honey and distillate preparation. Once we have corrected the malfunctions in the metabolism, you will be free of such symptoms as severe arthritis.

H

Halitosis: The state of having offensive breath; osostomia.

Remedy: Bad breath could be due to a number of causes. In what condition are your teeth? A periodic visit (every six months if possible or, at a minimum, at least once a year) to the dentist will be sufficient to take care of this concern. Two of the causes of bad breath are diet and problems with our digestive system. Similarly, the malfunctioning of certain glands may cause bad body odor. With the exception of the dentist's case, the other problems can be corrected or reduced by taking the Aloe, honey and distillate preparation. The preparation enables the body to perform its functions more efficiently because our body was created to function efficiently.

Hemorrhoids: A dilated and tortuous vein in the lower rectal or anal wall; a pile.

Remedy: Normally, one develops hemorrhoid problems as a result of constipation of the belly. Going to the bathroom is fundamental! Ideally, one should evacuate as many times a day as one eats. At a minimum, it is necessary to evacuate once a day. Twice a day, what a joy! Schedule going to the bathroom. Get the intestine used to this to avoid this pathology. However, when you have come down with the problem, what do you do? Turn to the Aloe, honey and distillate preparation. It will regulate the intestine.

To treat a severe case of hemorrhoids, make a suppository out of the gel in the Aloe leaf. Alternately, you can dampen a gauze, a cotton swab or a soft piece of cloth and apply it as you would a suppository. Do this in the evening before going to bed. In the morning, throw it out. Continue this treatment until

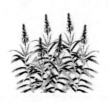

you have completely eliminated the problem. Do not stop after one or two treatments because you have seen improvements. It is important to attack the problem at the root, eliminating it totally.

Hepatitis: Inflammation of the liver.

Remedy: Currently, hepatitis A, hepatitis B, hepatitis C, hepatitis D, and hepatitis E exist. Since we are dealing with an inflammation of the liver, and more specifically of a viral nature, treat yourself with the Aloe, honey and distillate preparation. The liver is very receptive to an Aloe treatment.

Herpes: A spreading cutaneous infection. **Herpes simplex:** A viral disorder, characterized by groups of vesicles on an erythematous base. Commonly recurrent, and at times seen in the same place. **Herpes zoster:** An acute viral infectious disease of man, characterized by unilateral segmental inflammation of the posterior root ganglia and roots (and sometimes of anterior roots and posterior horn), or sensory ganglia of cranial nerves and by a painful vesicular eruption of the skin or mucous membranes in the peripheral distribution of the individual nerve or nerves.

Remedy: Because we are dealing with an infection, there is no better treatment than the Aloe, honey, and distillate

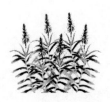

preparation. It is equally effective for the treatment of both herpes simplex and herpes zoster.

Hypertension: Excessive tension or pressure, especially that exerted by bodily fluids such as blood or aqueous humor. **Arterial hypertension:** Abnormally elevated blood pressure in the arterial side of the circulatory system. **Pseudo-tumor cerebri:** A syndrome of increased intracranial pressure associated with normal or small cerebral ventricles, of unknown etiology but, in children, sometimes associated with obstruction of the large intracranial sinuses or veins, particularly the lateral sinus. **Renovascular hypertension:** Systemic arterial hypertension as a result of intrinsic renal vascular disease; it is usually mediated through the renal pressor system.

Remedy: Finding the cause of the problem is a very wise approach. It should always be this way. In the case of hypertension, regardless of the type and of the affected organ, it is fundamental to know why the pressure exceeds 150/100 ml of mercury. Although we are not able to get to the cause of hypertension, let's make ourselves the Aloe, honey and distillate preparation. Once it has been determined that you have high blood pressure, who knows, maybe our preparation, once in the system, will be able to somehow distend or relax the overloaded organ, especially through the purification of the blood, and improve the flow of blood. How wonderful if you are able to get relief from your problem!

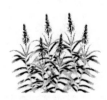

I

Indigestion: Inability to digest or difficulty in digesting something.

Remedy: The definition implies the presence of a system irregularity that impedes the proper execution of the digestive process. The abundant medicinal substances contained in the Aloe plant make it the right remedy for all types of irregularities of the digestive system. The recommended treatment is the Aloe, honey and distillate preparation. Of course, normally you would take the preparation before meals, but there is nothing wrong with taking a small amount after meals for the purpose of aiding digestion.

Infections: The invasion of a host by organisms such as bacteria, fungi, viruses, protozoa, helminths, or insects, with or without manifest disease.

Remedy: If the infection develops as a result of yeast, it does not matter whether it affects the bladder or the kidneys. All we need to know is that we are dealing with an infection. Such being the case, take the Aloe, honey and distillate preparation. In little time, the organs will be disinfected and restored to normal efficiency.

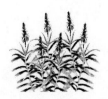

Ingrown toenails: Having the free tip or edge imbedded in the flesh.

Remedy: Oftentimes, ingrown toenails are removed with a scalpel. The topical application of the Aloe leaf would do away with surgery. The topical application is both painless and inexpensive.

Insomnia: Sleeplessness, disturbed sleep; prolonged inability to sleep.

Remedy: Here's the fundamental problem: why can't an individual fall asleep? Sleep is a vital necessity. The fact that we do not have sound information that sheds light on this matter, either in theory or in practice, should not stop you from beginning to solve it. So, make yourself the Aloe, honey and distillate preparation. It will not hurt. It is widely known that the plant contains soothing ingredients. Besides, it will also purify the body. Being intelligent, if the body thinks that it needs something, it will search for it in its constant attempt to always perform at optimal efficiency.

Intestinal parasites: Organisms that live, during part or all of its existence, on or in another organism, the host, at whose expense it obtains nourishment and, in some cases, other benefits necessary for survival. This condition is usually detrimental, though not normally fatal, to the host.

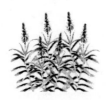

Remedy: To eliminate these intestinal parasites (found even in the nose, the bladder, or the rectum), we recommend a prolonged use of the Aloe, honey, and distillate preparation, anywhere from three to six months, and with brief intervals between jars (three to four days, or one week at the most). The prolonged treatment contributes to the total and definitive elimination of the parasite from the system by preventing its reproduction.

Irritation of the mouth: A normal or excessive reaction of the tissues to a specific stimulus. Irritation of the throat, the nasal mucosa, etc. Pathologically, an exacerbated reaction to a lesion; incipient inflammation.

Remedy: When we are dealing with irritation or, more precisely, inflammation, the Aloe, honey and distillate preparation is manna from the sky. It does not matter whether the irritation is in the mouth, in the throat, or in the mucosa. Work with Aloe!

Itching of any type: A sensation of tickling and irritation in the skin, producing a desire to scratch.

Remedy: It is important to determine the cause of the itch, just as it is for any abnormal condition. However, whether you know the cause of this sensation or not, turn to the Aloe, honey, and distillate preparation. Most likely, it's only a matter of

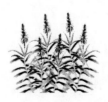

strengthening a weakened system. The preparation can help you. In addition to the preparation, another solution could be the topical application of the juice of the plant's leaf, even more so if the itching is temporary.

J

Jaundice: Yellow pigmentation of the skin and mucous membranes due to an excess of bilirubin and the deposition of bile pigments. These conditions are brought on by an accumulation of the hepatic cells (jaundice from hepatitis, cirrhosis, and from various types of intoxications), from the blockage of the extrahepatic bile tracts, and from the widespread destruction of the red blood cells (hemolysis).

Remedy: If it is true that jaundice is characterized by an accumulation of hepatic cells, by the obstruction of the bile tract and by the destruction of the red blood cells, let's shoot for a full recovery of the hepatic cells. Let's go and free the bile tract. Let's go and restore the destroyed red blood cells. Let's make the Aloe, honey and distillate preparation. Do not be surprised if your initiative pays off.

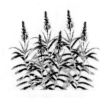

L

Laryngitis: Inflammation of the larynx. It may be acute or chronic, catarrhal, suppurative, croupous (diphtheritic), tuberculous, or syphilitic.

Remedy: Since we are dealing with the inflammation of the duct between the pharynx and the trachea located in the median and anterior part of the neck, turn to the Aloe, honey and distillate preparation for the solution. If you are left only with inflammation, consider this a small problem.

Leprosy: An infectious disease of low communicability, due to invasion of nerves by acid-fast Mycobacterium leprae; followed by progressive local invasion of tissues or hematogenous spread to skin, ciliary bodies, testes, lymph nodes, and nerves.

Remedy: Besides taking the Aloe, honey and distillate preparation without intervals, the patient can apply the pulpous part of the plant over the affected areas, keeping it there even for 24 hours, and substituting it with fresh pieces several times a day. Instead of the topical application, alternate the treatment with a fresh leaf or with a good quality Aloe-based ointment.

Leukemia: Any disease of the hemolytopoietic system characterized by uncontrolled proliferation of the leukocytes.

Anaplastic leukocytes usually are present in the blood, often in large numbers, and characteristically involve various organs. Leukemias are classified on the basis of rapidity of course (acute, subacute, or chronic), the cell count, the cell type and the degree of differentiation.

Remedy: If we had a list of all the different types of tumors Aloe has cured, I am certain that we would find leukemia at the very top of the list.

It is sufficient to use the Aloe, honey and distillate preparation. This preparation interrupts the uncontrolled proliferation of the white blood cells, and promotes the development of healthy cells. There is no need for a marrow transplant (donor compatible), nor for radiation treatments or chemotherapy. The simple truth is that the preparation has re-established order in that body. The patient should undergo medical examinations.

Lupus: Any chronic progressive ulcerative skin lesion. **Lupus erythematosus:** A disease of unknown cause and variable manifestations, ranging from a skin disorder (discoid lupus erythematosus) to a generalized disorder involving the skin and viscera (systemic lupus erythematosus).

Remedy: Treat this illness the same as you would leprosy, with the Aloe, honey and distillate preparation taken orally. Relative to the ulcerations, apply the pulp part of a fresh leaf, substituting it two or three times a day, or alternating with a

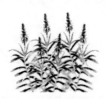

good quality Aloe-based ointment. Total cure is relatively fast, though it varies from individual to individual. We recommend the patient undergo a physician's evaluation to show improvements obtained.

M

Mastitis (in cows): Any inflammatory infection of the mammary gland.

Aloe is also very beneficial to animals. It can be used on cows, dogs, horses, pigs, cats, etc. In the case of mastitis, turn to a topical application. The animal's owner should bear in mind that an animal is positively sensitive to hygiene and it responds favorably when you take good care of it.

Meningitis: Any inflammation of the membranes of the brain or spinal cord. Meningitis may be classified according to the causative agent as tuberculous meningitis or pneumococcal meningitis.

Remedy: If we are dealing with an inflammation of the meninx and its source is bacterial, toxic, or parasitic, turn to the Aloe, honey, and distillate preparation, an excellent remedy for these cases. The preparation should be taken as soon as the symptoms are noticed to help the patient's immune system right from the outset. The sooner the treatment is started, the

better the chances of eliminating or minimizing the consequences of the illness.

Migraine: Recurrent paroxysmal vascular headache; varying in
intensity, frequency, and duration; commonly unilateral in
onset and often associated with nausea and vomiting; may be
preceded by or associated with sensory, motor, or mood
disturbances; often familial.

   Remedy: It is also widely accepted that the cause for the
headache is unknown. If it is not known, it's because it's not
worth knowing! It is as clear as daylight that such a painful
condition originates from digestive problems, caused by an
inadequate diet. Don't pay attention to that idle talk. Turn to the
Aloe, honey and distillate preparation. After approximately one
week, you will experience noticeable improvements. Continue
your treatment. After two or three jars of the preparation, your
migraines will be a thing of the past.

Multiple sclerosis: Multiple sclerosis equals plaque in the
muscles. A common disease of young adults, characterized
clinically by episodes of focal disorder of the optic nerves,
spinal cord, and brain, which remit to a varying extent and
recur over a period of many years, and pathologically by the
presence of numerous, scattered, sharply defined demyelinative
lesions (plaques) in the white matter of the central nervous
system.

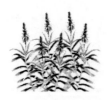

Remedy: To beat this terrifying disease, plan on taking the Aloe, honey, and distillate preparation for a period of anywhere from three to six months continuously (if you take a break between jars, make sure it isn't longer than three or four days, a week at the very most). Such therapy can restore the body's normal activities. Even though we are dealing with a number of pathologies, you will notice that the recurrence of multiple sclerosis will be considerably reduced.

Muscle cramp: A painful involuntary spasmodic contraction of a muscle. A temporary paralysis of muscles from overuse.

Remedy: Such contraction is probably brought on by insufficient oxygen in the muscle. Take the Aloe, honey and distillate to permeate the blood vessels.

You can avoid this problem by eating one banana a day.

Myopia: Nearsightdness; an optical defect, usually due to too great a length of the anteroposterior diameter of the globe, whereby the focal image is formed in front of the retina. The opposite of myopia is:

Hyperopia (farsightdness): A refractive error in which, with suspended accommodation, the focus of parallel rays of light falls behind the retina; due to an abnormally short antero-posterior diameter of the eye or to subnormal refractive power.

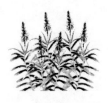

Presbyopia: The condition of vision commonly seen after the middle forties but beginning in late childhood (after age 8), due to diminished power of accommodation from impaired elasticity of the crystalline lens, whereby the near point of distinct vision is removed farther from the eye, so that the individual has difficulties in focusing on near objects and in reading fine print.

Remedy: After taking the Aloe, honey, and distillate preparation for a few months, people who used to use eyeglasses to read, to their disbelief, slowly find they can do without them. Since there are no side effects, take this preparation regularly. This is especially recommended for older people.

N

Nausea of any type: A feeling of discomfort in the region of the stomach, with aversion to food and a tendency to vomit.

Remedy: The dictionary's definition does not help us learn the source of nausea. It is probably due to some kind of liver, stomach or pancreas malfunction. In short, a malfunction of the digestive apparatus. To free yourself of nausea, all you need is to put a little piece of the Aloe leaf in your mouth. In a very short time, you either vomit or expel the foreign body that was

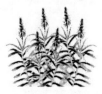

the cause of this problem. Begin taking the Aloe, honey, and distillate preparation regularly in order to avoid these types of problems in the future.

Obesity: An increase in body weight due to an accumulation of fat, 10 to 20 percent beyond the normal range for the particular age, sex, and height. It can be **ectogenous**, due to an excessively abundant diet, or **endogenous**, due to metabolic or endocrine dysfunctions.

   Remedy: If the accumulation of fat is due to an excessively rich diet, practice better self-control: shut your mouth! Advise a lady to see a doctor if she is worried about a weight increase. If the problem arises from metabolic or endocrine dysfunctions, a good specialist in the field would be the patient's best choice.

   Beware of miraculous diets: they promise miracles! Today we have the NUTRACEUTICA, the new nutrition science. It promises miracles in this field. Time will tell. In the meantime, while we wait for miracles, turn to the Aloe, honey, and distillate preparation; it may be able the restore metabolism and glands to their normal function.

Odor (bad, caused by ulcers): The characteristic of some bodies to emanate volatile particles that are able to stimulate the

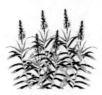

olfactory organs of man and of some animals, and is perceived in diverse sensations; odor (strong, imperceptible, inebriating, nauseating).

Remedy: Surely the odor that some bodies give off must be attributed to the anomalous functioning of the glands responsible for its release. Let's turn to the Aloe, honey, and distillate preparation to help restore order to the entire system. You can also turn to topical application. Blend an Aloe leaf and use the resultant mixture, by itself or mixed with water, as a cleanser. Wash the body parts, leaving it to dry on the body. When finished, have a shower.

P

Pancreatitis (pancreatic problems): Inflammation of the pancreas, acute or chronic.

Remedy: As the term implies, we are dealing with the inflammation of the abdominal gland. Therefore, get to a jar of Aloe, honey, and distillate preparation. The Aloe will aid the production of higher quality pancreatic juice that subsequently makes its way to the duodenum. This is very important because, with its higher enzyme content, the pancreatic juice greatly facilitates the digestion process.

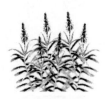

Prostatitis/Prostatism: Prostatitis: Inflammation of the prostate gland. **Prostatism:** the condition caused by chronic disorders of the prostate, especially obstruction of urination by prostatic enlargement.

Remedy: Just as in the case of leukemia, if we had statistics on the success rate of the Aloe, honey, and distillate preparation for curing illnesses, we have reason to believe that prostatic problems would be at the very top of the list, probably immediately below leukemia. It really works! Do not waste time! Turn to the Aloe preparation at once.

Psoriasis: An idiopathic chronic inflammatory skin disease characterized by the development of red patches covered with silvery-white imbricated scales. The disease affects especially the extensor surfaces of the body and the scalp.

Remedy: Because it has to do with the inflammation of the skin, do a lupus-style topical application. Also, use the Aloe, honey, and distillate preparation, which will free the system of the toxins responsible for the plaques located in specific areas of the body. The standard treatments administered up to the present by traditional medicine, including the mud from the Dead Sea, are nothing but palliatives. A true cure has only happened in Saudi Arabia, about June of 1996, when Dr. Syed demonstrated, unequivocally, the healing qualities of Aloe on psoriasis. His study lasted 16 weeks. He applied an Aloe

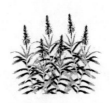

ointment on 36 patients, and 25 of them were completely cured of the illness. Why don't they continue with similar experiences? The reader, being intelligent, knows the reasons.

R

Rough hands: None of the dictionaries that I have consulted gives a definition of this pathology, if we can even refer to it as a pathology.

    Remedy: To the person who lives with this problem, I would recommend taking the Aloe, honey, and distillate preparation. To speed up the process, I would supplement that with topical application of the Aloe leaf's juice. Of course, such application is not to be limited to a case of rough hands only; it can be extended to our entire skin, our main organ. The reaction will be fast.

S

Sciatica: Pain along the course of the sciatic nerve, caused by inflammation or injury to the nerve or its roots, and most commonly due to a herniated disk of the lower lumbar or upper sacral spine. In addition to the pain, there is numbness, tingling,

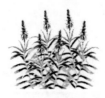

and tenderness along the course of the nerve, and eventually loss of the ankle jerk and superficial sensation in the distribution of the involved root or roots.

Remedy: Turn to the Aloe, honey, and distillate preparation. Since Aloe is an excellent analgesic, at a minimum it will provide you with relief from the pain. You will experience relief in a matter of days after beginning this treatment. In addition, do not forget that Aloe is a lubricant.

Seborrhoea: A functional disease of the sebaceous glands, characterized by an excessive secretion or disturbed quality of sebum, which collects upon the skin in the form of an oily coating or of crusts or scales.

Remedy: The Aloe, honey, and distillate preparation will free the sebaceous glands, allowing the secretion, up to now restricted, to resume its regular flow through the normal excretion ducts.

Sinusitis: Inflammation of a sinus. May affect any of the paranasal sinuses, as ethmoidal, frontal, maxillary, or sphenoid.

Remedy: Enough with suffering! Do away with the old pains that come from sinusitis. Take the Aloe, honey, and distillate preparation and you will solve your problems. It works wonders! Do not be surprised at the amount of toxins

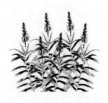

and waste that will be expelled. However, expect a long healing process.

Sprain: A wrenching of a joint, producing a stretching or laceration of the ligaments.

Remedy: Turn to topical application. Massage the traumatized area very gently. Thanks to a fast penetration of its gel into the skin, the Aloe, with its potent analgesic properties, will give you immediate relief from the pain.

Sterility due to anovular cycles: Total inability to reproduce.

Remedy: There are so many cases of married couples who have long desired a child but, in their many attempts, have been unsuccessful in conceiving one. Quite a large number of people have even attempted artificial insemination, as well as other means, some of them painful and all in vain. Over the years, I have advised couples to take the Aloe, honey, and distillate preparation for three consecutive months for a purification of the system. Only afterwards can they attempt to reproduce again. The first couple I advised came from Rome, Italy. The couple confided their problem to me in Bethlehem in 1993, when I was stationed in the Holy Land. Today, at Porto Alegre alone there must be half a dozen "Aloe children," as they are affectionately called. The fortunate couples are the first to acknowledge that it was the Aloe preparation that precipitated

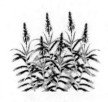

the process of their happiness, from frustration to a state of total fulfilment as parents.

What is Aloe's role? It unblocks all the involved tracts so nature can take its course.

Stiff neck (Torticollis): Deformity of the neck due to contraction of cervical muscles or fascia, but mostly involving the sternocleidomastoid muscle unilaterally, resulting in abnormal position and limitation of movements of the head.

Remedy: One of the factors that could bring this condition about is temperature contrast: going from the warmth of the bathroom to the coolness of the corridor, or exposure to a draught.

To resolve this problem, grind one or two Aloe leaves to make a poultice. Apply this poultice to the affected area and massage it lightly. Then raise the body temperature by putting on additional clothing. What relief you will experience! You have resolved the problem.

Stings (scorpion, spider, cobra, insects: bee, gnat, fly, etc.): The acute burning sensation caused by pricking, striking, or chemically stimulating the skin or a mucous membrane.

Remedy: Immediately apply a topical application of the internal (gelatinous) part of the Aloe leaf over the cutaneous lesions caused by the insect. Bandage it and leave it there from

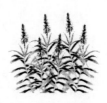

40 minutes to one hour. Replace it more often if you are dealing with the bite of a poisonous cobra. Speaking of a cobra's bite, when you remove the bandage, observe the change in color of the pulpous part of the Aloe leaf that you used over the wound. That is evidence that the poison has been extracted from the wound. Therefore, consider this a successful first aid treatment, especially if you have been unable to get to a hospital. At the first opportunity, however, see to it that you get to a hospital for an antiophidic serum treatment.

Stomach acid (acidity, gastritis, gastric hyperacidity, pyrosis): Pyrosis: a substernal or epigastric burning sensation accompanied by eructation of an acrid, irritating fluid; heartburn.

Remedy: In such cases (acidity, gastritis, inflammation), can one use Aloe? If yes, how?

Put together a complete recipe of Aloe, honey and distillate. A jar will solve the problem. To confirm its positive results, take a second jar and, eventually, even a third, without long intervals between them (three or four days, one week at the most).

Alternate option: keep a tablet of natural Aloe in your mouth all day, swallowing the saliva.

A different form: cut the leaf into pieces, as you would with an onion. Put it in water and drink it. Add more water and, an

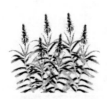

hour or two later, drink that, too. Continue doing this for the entire day.

T

Tendonitis: Inflammation of a tendon, usually at the point of its attachment to bone.

Remedy: You are an expert by now. As soon as you realize that you are dealing with an inflammation, turn to the Aloe, honey, and distillate preparation. It can resolve the problem. If the tendonitis has been caused by a trauma, the topical application is also recommended. If, on the other hand, it proceeds from a degenerative cause, then make use of the preparation only.

Tonsillitis: Inflammation of the tonsils.

Remedy: As the definition states, we are dealing with an inflammation of the tonsils. Because it is a localized inflammation, the solution is the Aloe, honey, and distillate preparation.

Note: If you desire, you may also keep a small, rectangular piece of Aloe leaf in your mouth as if it were a chewing gum, and only swallow the saliva that will be secreted. You can do

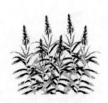

this both during the day as well as at night. Such continuous therapy will speed up the disinfection process.

Trachoma: An infectious disease of the conjunctiva and cornea, producing photophobia, pain, excessive tearing, and sometimes blindness, caused by **Chlamydia trachomatis**. The lesion is characterized initially by inflammation and later by pannus and follicular and papillary hypertrophy of the conjunctiva. **Pannus:** Vascularization and connective-tissue deposition beneath the epithelium of the cornea.

    Remedy: Turn to the two possible therapies: topical and internal. Apply one drop of the juice from an Aloe leaf several times a day. Because we are dealing with an inflammation caused by **Chlamydia trachomatis** – next of kin to a virus – turn to the Aloe, honey, and distillate preparation in an effort to dislodge it from its hideout. With the preparation, we will purify the entire system.

Tuberculosis: A chronic infectious disease with protean manifestation, primarily involving the lungs, but capable of attacking most organs of the body, caused by **Mycobacterium tuberculosis**. Usually the primary infection is stopped, but widespread tuberculous disease occasionally occurs. Severe clinical manifestations may include fever, weight loss, cough, chest pain, sputum, and hemoptysis. The pathological response may include tubercle formation, exudation, necrosis, and fibrosis,

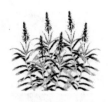

depending on local biochemical factors, the hypersensitive state, the number and virulence of the organisms, and the resistance of the host. Abbreviated TB.

Remedy: On page 67 of his book **The Curative Power of the Aloe (O poder curative da babosa)**, Neil Stevens says: "Research on tuberculosis conducted by Doctor Ghottshall, et al. in 1950 already pointed to the enormous potential of Aloe as a remedy for respiratory ailments."

Turn to the Aloe, honey, and distillate preparation as a defense against the disease, which was the terror of the 1950s and that today is making a return, just when it seemed it had been wiped out. Take Aloe and you will win the battle! Follow up with medical examinations as well. If you want, you can take a short break between jars. Fight this dreadful illness without giving it a moment's respite.

U

Ulcer *(Duodenal, peptic, stasis, in general):* An interruption of continuity of an epithelial surface, with an inflamed base.

I'm including more types of ulcers so we can better understand the subject matter. **Atonic ulcer:** An indolent or slow-healing ulcer. **Bauru ulcer:** A skin ulcer occurring in *American mucocutaneous leishmaniasis.* **Decubitus ulcer:** Ulceration of the skin and subcutaneous tissues due to protein defici-

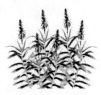

ency and prolonged unrelieved pressure on bony prominences; seen commonly in aged, bedridden people. **Stercoraceous ulcer**: An ulcer of the skin is contaminated by feces. **Phagedena ulcer**: A rapidly spreading destructive ulceration of soft parts. **Peptic ulcer**: A sharp circumscribed loss of tissue, involving chiefly the mucosa, submucosa, and muscular layer in areas of the digestive tract exposed to acid-pepsin gastric juice, particularly the lower esophagus, stomach, and first portion of the duodenum. **Mal perforant**: Perforating ulcer of the foot. **Stasis ulcer**: Ulceration, usually of the leg, due to chronic venous insufficiency or venous stasis.

Remedy: As already stated, it is fundamental to treat any type of ulcer with the Aloe, honey, and distillate preparation with the specific objective of purifying the system. In the case of an exposed, open ulcer such as a decubitus ulcer, turn to the topical application of the Aloe leaf either in ground form or cut into small pieces. Prepare the poultice and apply it over the wound, repeating the treatment three times a day with a fresh poultice each time. You'll save money, and with 100% efficiency.

Urticaria: Hives or nettle rash. A skin condition characterized by the appearance of intensely itching wheals or welts with elevated, usually white, centers and a surrounding area of erythema. They tend to disappear in a day or two, and usually are unattended by constitutional symptoms.

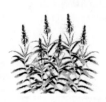

Remedy: By now you're an expert! You know we are dealing with a case of infection and, for this condition, you should turn to the Aloe, honey, and distillate preparation. The topical application of the gel contained inside the plant's leaf may speed up the process of eliminating these papules from the skin. However, if you experience itching or irritation, stop the topical application and continue with the oral preparation treatment only.

V

Vaginitis: Inflammation of the vagina.

Remedy: Because we are dealing with an inflammation, quickly turn to the Aloe, honey, and distillate preparation. If there are any irregularities in your system, this preparation will set it straight. The topical application of the gel of a liquefied leaf will give immediate benefits.

Varix: 1. A dilated and torturous vein. 2. A torturous, enlarged artery or lymphatic vessel.

Remedy: The dilation of a vein is probably due to either poor blood circulation or poor blood quality. If this is the case, let's try to purify the blood and its circulation. If the problem is of a different nature, the Aloe, honey, and distillate preparation will help the body find a solution to the problem. The topical application of the pulp of the Aloe leaf, without the removal of its skin, is also recommended.

Weakness: The quality or state of lacking strength, of being physically deficient, of not being able to resist external force or withstand attack, of feeling feeble, debilitated.

Remedy: The definition clearly depicts the state of health of the patient. The Aloe, honey and distillate preparation will assist a person in this state. Aloe, with its more than 300 useful substances, all important and essential for your body, will help you get out of the bottom of the well. Once outside, take care of yourself so you won't fall back in again. Take care of your health!

Wounds of all types: The disruption of normal anatomical relationships, or loss of tissue, resulting from surgery or physical injury. Lesions produced in the skin or in the mucosa by a blow or impact from a rigid object of a sharp or perforating nature; injuring; by extension, open lesions with loss of fluid; sores, ulcers, wounding.

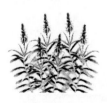

Remedy: The wound produced in the skin or in the mucosa, accompanied at times with loss of blood due to the violence of the impact suffered, demands immediate topical application of Aloe. It is a first aid remedy; it should be among all the first aid remedies within reach of people involved in accidents.

However, when you are dealing with an open wound, one with suppuration – an old wound – the best remedy is the Aloe, honey and distillate preparation, since such a wound is difficult to heal due to the blood's poor quality. However, the simultaneous topical application of the gelatinous part of the leaf over the affected area will promote a faster healing process.

Z

Zoster: See Herpes.

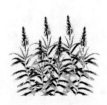

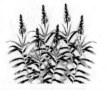

Afterward

As you can see, in **Aloe isn't medicine, and Yet...It Cures!**, we have thought of placing this booklet in the hands of the less fortunate with the hope that it may help them overcome some of the difficulties that life, at times unexpectedly, serves all of us with. Our objective is to help these people to contend with these difficulties, offering them our experiences. How nice it would be if our remedy resolved the problem!

It would be foolish to think that, by presenting Aloe as a medical remedy, we don't give any merit to or, even worse, disdain traditional medicine. It would be a ridiculous view!

Our intent is to offer the less fortunate assistance to overcome the limitations brought on by a challenging reality. The Aloe, honey, and distillate preparation is to be interpreted as an alternative solution to their problem. Have we been successful? I pray to God we have!

We wish that one day all citizens of the world, with equal rights and duties, will have access to all the resources, including access to good health, that God has made available to all His creatures, so they may live a dignified life.

If, by chance, you have utilized Aloe to fight a type of illness that we haven't listed in this book and you would like to tell us about it, please write to us and include in your correspondence

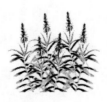

your personal identification data and how we can contact you along with the following information:

- the name of the illness treated;
- how you have employed Aloe (internal or external use);
- the outcome.

It will be our pleasure to relate your case in eventual subsequent editions so that others who find themselves facing the same difficult situation, may economically and effectively benefit from your experience. All very fraternally, my friend.

You can contact us by post or e-mail as follows:

Fr. Romano Zago, OFM
Caixa Postal 2330
90001-970 Porto Alegre, RS-Brazil
Email: freiromanozago@bol.com.br

The author

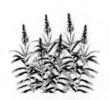

Bibliography, including Specific International Journals

Acevedo-Duncan, M., Russell, C., Patel, S., Patel, R.: Aloe-emodin-modulates PKC isozymes, inhibits proliferation, and induces apoptosis in U-373MG glioma cella. International Immuno-pharmacology 4(14):1775-1784., 2004.

Afzal, M., Ali, M., Hassan, R.A.H., Sweedan, N., Dhami, M.S.I.: Identification of some prostanoids in Aloe vera extracts. Planta Medica 57, 38-40, 1991.

Ando, N., Yamaguchi, I.: Sitosterol from Aloe vera gel. Kenkyu Kiyo-Tokyo Kasei Daigaku 30, 1520, 1990.

Anton, R., Haag-Berrurier, M.: Therapeutic use of natural anthraquinone for other than laxative actions. Pharmacology 20, 104-112, 1980.

Ashley, F.L, O'Loughlin, B.J., Peterson, R., Fernandez, L., Stein, H., Schwartz, A.N.: The use of Aloe vera in the treatment of thermal and irradiation burns in laboratory animals and humans. Plastic and Reconstructive Surgery 20, 383-396, 1957.

Avila, H., Rivero, J., Herrera, F., Fraile, G.: Cytotoxicity of a low molecular weight fraction from Aloe vera (Aloe barbadensis Miller) gel. Toxicon 35, 1423-1430, 1997.

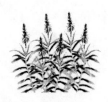

Azghani, A.O., Williams, I., Holiday, D.B., Johnson, A.R.: A betalinked mannan inhibits adherence of Pseudomonas aeruginosa to human lung epithelial cells. Glycobiology 5, 39-44, 1995.

Basso, G., Diaspro, A., Salvato, B., Carli, M., Palu, G.: Aloe-emodin is a new type of anticancer agent with selective activity against neuroectodermal tumors. Cancer Research 60(11):2800-2804, 2000.

Beppu, H., Koitz, T., Shimpo, K., Chihara, T., Hoshino, M., Ida, C., Kuzuya, H.: Radical-scavenging effect of <u>Aloe arborescens</u> Miller on prevention of pancreatic islet B-cell destruction in rats. Journal of Ethnopharmacology, 89 (1):27-45, 2003.

Beppu, H., Shimpo, K., Chihara, T., Kaneko, T., Tamai, I., Yamaji, S., Ozaki, S., Kuzuya, H., Sonoda, S.: Fujita Memorial Nanakuri Institute, Fujita Health University, 1865 Isshiki-cho, Hisai, Mie 514-1296, Japan. Anti-diabetic effects of dietary administration of <u>Aloe arborescens</u> Miller components on multiple low-dose streptozotocin-induced diabetes in mice: investigation on hypoglycemic action and systemic absorption dynamics of aloe components. J Ethnopharmacol. 103(3):468-77, 2006 Feb 20.

Bland, J.: Effect of orally consumed Aloe vera juice on gastro-intestinal function in normal humans. Linus Pauling Institute of Science & Medicine, Palo Alto, California, Preventive Medicine 14, 152-154, 1985.

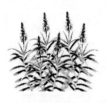

Blitz, J., Smith, J.W., Gerard, J.R.: Aloe vera gel in peptic ulcer therapy: preliminary report. Journal of the American Osteopathic Association 62, 731-735, 1963.

Boertman J.A.; Smith, D.J., Jr.; Sachs, R.J.: Experimental and Clinical Observations on Frostbite, Ann Emerg Med Sep 16 (9) 1056-62, 1987

Bloomfield, F.: Miracle Plants: Aloe Vera. Century, London, 1985.

Brossat, J.Y., Ledeaut, J.Y., Ralamboranto, L., Rakotovao, L.H., Solar, S., Gueguen, A., Coulanges, P.: Immuno-stimulating properties of an extract isolated from Aloe vahombe. Archives Institut Pasteur Madagascar 48, 11-34, 1981.

Bruce, W.G.G.: Investigations of antibacterial activity in the Aloe. South African Medical Journal 41, 984, 1967.

Bruce, W.G.G.: Medicinal properties in the Aloe. Excelsa 57-68, 1975.

Bunyapraphatsara et al.: The Benefits of Aloe Vera Juice on Diabetes, Phytomedicine (1996). Vol. 3(3), pp. 245-8

Capasso, F., Borrelli, F., Capasso, R., DiCarlo, G., Izzo, A.A., Pinto, L., Mascolo, N., Castaldo, S., Longo, R.: Aloe and its therapeutic use. Phytotherapy Research 12, S124-S127, 1998. Special Issue: Proceedings of the Second International Symposium on Natural Drugs, Maratea, Italy, September 28-

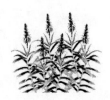

October 1, 1997. Published Online: 18 Dec 1998, © 2008 John Wiley & Sons, Ltd.: ABSTRACT: Aloe is one of the few medicinal plants that has maintained its popularity for a long period of time. Aloe latex is used for its laxative effect and should be distinguished from aloe gel, used both in cosmetics and ointments for skin ailments. Aloe whole leaf is another preparation used internally as a drink in a wide range of human diseases including cancer, AIDS, ulcerative colitis and other disturbances. The concomitant use of honey may make the aloe whole leaf therapy more palatable and efficient. © 1998 John Wiley & Sons, Ltd.

Cera, L.M., Heggers, J.P., Robson, M.C., Hagstrom, W.J.: The therapeutic efficacy of Aloe vera cream (Dermaide Aloe™) in thermal injuries. Two case reports. J. Am. Animal Hospital Assoc. 16, 768-772, 1980.

Chikalo, I., Bolovyeve, V., Ukraine, The Small Intestines' Function Affected by Aloe Extract, quoted in "The Aloes of Tropical Africa and Madagascar," by Reynolds, G.W., Sept. 1966

Coats, Bill C., R.Ph., C.C.N., with Ahola, Robert: Aloe Vera, the New Millennium, i Universe, 2003.

Danhof, Ivan E., M.D., Ph.D., (ND): The Fundamentals of Aloe Vera Mucopolysaccharides. Abstract: Dr. Danhof is regarded by many as the leading authority on the Aloe vera plant. This

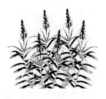

paper gives the fundamentals of how the polysaccharide molecules help the body in the healing process, 1994.

Danhof, Ivan E., M.D., Ph.D, (ND): Aloe Vera Leaf Handling and Constituent Variability; Remarkable Aloe – Aloe Through the Ages, Vol. 1, Omnimedicus Press, 1987.

Danhof, Ivan E, M.D., Ph.D.: Internal uses of Aloe vera. Abstract: Aloe used in intestinal disorders, atherosclerosis and coronary hearth disease, anti-cancer actions, immunity, 1988.

Danhof, Ivan E., M.D., Ph.D.: Aloe Vera, The Whole Leaf Advantage, Private Paper, North Texas Research Laboratory, 2000

Danhof, Ivan E., M.D., Ph.D.: New Approach in the Treatment of Diabetic Foot Ulcers, Private Paper, North Texas Research Laboratory, 2000

Danhof, Ivan E., M.D., Ph.D.: The Antitumor Effects of Aloe Vera? North Texas Research Laboratory. Omnimedicus Press. Grand Prairie, Texas. 2000

Davis, R.H.: Topical influence of Aloe vera on adjuvant arthritis, inflammation and wound healing. Physiologist 31, 206, 1988.

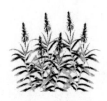

Davis, R.H., Agnew, P.S., Shapiro, E.: Anti-arthritic activity of anthraquinones found in Aloe for podiatric medicine. Journal of the American Podiatric Medical Association 76, 61-66, 1986.

Davis, R.H., Kabbani, J.M., Maro, N.P.: Wound healing and anti-inflammatory activity of Aloe vera. Proceedings of the Pennsylvania Academy of Science 60, 79, 1986.

Davis, R.H., Leitner, M.G., Russo, J.: Topical anti-inflammatory activity of Aloe vera as measured by ear swelling. Journal of the American Podiatric Medical Association 77, 610-612, 1987.

Davis, R.H., Leitner, M.G., Russo, J.M., Byrne, M.E.: Anti-inflammatory activity of Aloe vera against a spectrum of irritants. Journal of the American Podiatric Medical Association 79, 263-276, 1989.

Davis, R.H., Maro, N.P.: Aloe vera and gibberellin. Anti-inflammatory activity in diabetes. Journal of the American Podiatric Medical Association 79, 24-26, 1989.

Davis, Robert H., Ph.D., Professor Emeritus of Physiology: The Conductor-Orchestra Concept Of Aloe Vera, Aloe Vera/A Scientific Study. Vantage Press. New York. 1997. pp. 290-310

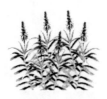

Davis, Robert H., Ph.D.; Leitner, Mark G.; Russo, Joseph M., B.A.: Aloe vera: A Natural Approach for Treating Wounds, Edema, and Pain Diabetes, Journal of the American Podiatric Medical Association Volume 78, Number 2, February 1988

Davis, Robert H., Ph.D.: Does Aloe Vera have a Place in AIDS Therapy?" Aloe Vera/A Scientic Approach., Vantage Press, New York, 1997

Davis, Robert H., Ph.D.: Biological Activity of Aloe Vera.

Davis, Robert H., Ph.D.; Parker, William L., B.A.; Samson, Richard T., B.S.; Murdoch, Douglas P.: The Isolation of an Active Inhibitory System from an Extract of Aloe vera, B.Sc American Podiatric Medical Association Volume 81, Number 5, May 1991

Davis, Robert H., Ph.D.; Joseph J. DiDonato B.S.: Aloe Vera Open Wound Healing Micro-Assay, Pennsylvania College of Podiatric Medicine, Philadelphia, Pennsylvania 19107

Duke, J.A.: Aloe barbadensis Mill. (Liliaceae). CRC Handbook of Medicinal Herbs. CRC Press, Boca Raton, FL, pp. 31-32, 1985.

Egger, S., Brown, G.S., Kelsey, L.S., Yates, K.M., Rosenberg, L.J., Talmadge, J.E.: Hematopoietic augmentation by a beta-(1,4)-linked mannan. Cancer Immunology Immuno-therapy 43, 195-205, 1996.

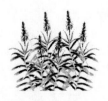

Elkins, Rita, M.H.: Miracle Sugars, The Glyconutrient Link to Disease Prevention and Improved Health, Woodland Publishing, 2003

Finbar, Magee (Dr.): Health watch: Alternative path: Aloe, aloe what's all this then? The News Letter. Belfast, Northern Ireland. Abstract: Lists some of the benefits of Aloe and also some of the 75 plus nutritional substances. "What is also apparent is that the plant itself is better than the sum of the individual components. In some way the synergistic balance out performs isolated components." (2002, November 6).

Frumkin, A.: Aloe vera, salicylic acid and aspirin for burns. Plastic and Reconstructive Surgery 83, 196, 1989.

Fujita, K., Ito, S., Teradaira, R., Beppu, H.: Properties of a carboxypeptidase from Aloe. Biochemical Pharmacology 28, 1261-1262, 1979.

Fujita, K., Yamada, Y., Azuma, K., Hirozawa, S.: Effect of leaf extracts of <u>Aloe arborescens</u> Mill subsp. natalensis Berger on growth of Trichophyton entagrophytes. Anti-microbial Agents and Chemotherapy 35, 132-136, 1978.

Furukawa, F., Nishikawa, A., Chihara, T., Shimpo, K., Beppu, H., Kuzuya, H., Lee, I.S., Hirosr, M.: Chemopreventive effects of <u>Aloe arborescens</u> on N-nitrosobis(2-oxopropyl) amine-induced pancreatic carcinogenesis in hamsters. Cancer Letters 178(2): 117-122, 2002.

Gardiner, T.: Biological Activity of eight known dietary mono-saccharides required for glycoprotein synthesis and cellular recognition processes: summary, Glyco Science & Nutrition 1(13):1-4, 2000.

Gauntt, C., et al.: Aloe polymannose enhances anti-coxsackievirus antibody titres in mice, Phytotherapy Research, 14(4):261-6, 2000 June.

Gowda, D.C., Neelisiddaiah, B., Anjaneyalu, Y.V.: Structural studies of polysaccharides from Aloe vera. Carbohydrate Research 72, 201-205, 1979.

Gribel, N.V.; Pashinskii, V.G.: Vopr Onkol 32(12):38-40 1986. An evaluation of antimetastatic properties of succus Aloes was carried out using three types of experimental tumors of mice and rats. It was found that succus Aloes treatment contributes to reduction of tumor mass, metastatic foci and metastasis frequency at different stages of tumor progress without affecting major tumor growth. Succus Aloes potentiates the anti-tumor effect of 5-fluorouracil and cyclophosphamide as components of combination chemotherapy.

Grindlay, D., Reynolds, T.: The Aloe vera phenomenon: a review of the properties and modern uses of the leaf parenchyma gel. Journal of Ethnopharmacology 16, 117-151, 1986.

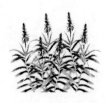

Haq, Q.N., Hannan, A.: Studies on glucogalactomannan from the leaves of Aloe vera, Tourn. (ex Linn.). Bangladesh Journal of Scientific and Industrial Research 16, 68-72, 1981.

Heggers, J.P., Kucukcelibi, A., Listengarten, D., Stabenau, C.J., Ko, F., Broemeling, L.D., Robson, M.C., Winters, W.D.: Beneficial effect of Aloe on wound healing in an excisional wound model. Journal of Alternative and Complementary Medicine 2, 271-277, 1996.

Heggers, J.P., Pelley, R.P., Robson, M.C.: Beneficial effects of Aloe in wound healing. Phytotherapy Research 7, S48-S52, 1993.

Hirata, T. & Suga T.: Aloenin and Aloe-Ulcin from <u>Aloe arborescens</u> Inhibit Gastric Secretion, J.Med. Soc. Toho Jpn. 17 361, 1970

Hiroko, Saito: Aloe's Effectiveness as an Anti-Inflammatory Agent, Department Of Pharmacy, Aichi Cancer Center, 1993

Hu, Y., Xu, J., Hu, Q.: Evaluation of antioxidant potential of aloe vera (Aloe barbadensis Miller) extracts. Journal of Agricultural and Food Chemistry 51(26):7788-7791, 2003.

Hutter, J.A., Salman, M., Stavinoha, W.B., Satsangi, N., Williams, R.F., Streeper, R.T., Weintraub, S.T.: Anti-inflammatory glucosyl chromone from Aloe barbadensis. Journal of Natural Products 59, 541-543, 1996.

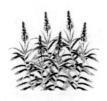

Imanishi, K.: Aloctin A, an active substance of <u>Aloe arborescens</u> Miller as an immunomodulator. Phytotherapy Research 7, S20-S22, 1993.

Jamieson, G.I.: Aloe vera (Aloe barbadensis Mill.). Queensland Agricultural Journal 110, 220, 1984.

Jeong, H.Y.; Kim, J.H.; Hwang, S.J.; Rhee, D.K.: Anticancer effects of Aloe on sarcoma 180 in ICR mouse or human cancer cells were determined. Sarcoma 180 cells were inoculated subcutaneously into male ICR mouse to determine effect of Aloe on tumor growth, or inoculated intraperitoneally into male ICR mouse to determine effect of Aloe on life span prolongation, followed by oral administration of Aloe vera (10 mg/kg/day, 50 mg/kg/day) or <u>Aloe arborescens</u> (10 mg/kg/day, 100 mg/kg/day) once a day for 14 days. Coll. Pharm., Sung Kyun Kwan Univ.Yakhak Hoeji 38 (3). 1994. 311-321

Kaufman, T., M.D.; Newman, A.R., M.D.; Wexler, M.R., M.D.: Aloe Vera and Burn Wound Healing, Department of Plastic Surgery and Burn Unit, Hadassah University Hospital, Ein Kerem, Jerusalem, Israel, June, 1989.

Kinoshita, K., Koyama, K., Takahashi, K., Noguchi, Y., Amano, M.: Steroid glucosides from Aloe barbadensis. Journal of Japanese Botany 71, 83-86, 1996.

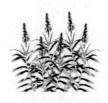

Kodym, A.: The main chemical components contained in fresh leaves and in a dry extract from three years old <u>Aloe arborescens</u> Mill. grown in hothouses. Pharmazie 46, 217-219, 1991.

Kodym, A., Marcinkowski, A., Kukula, H., Department of Drug Form Technology, Ludwik Rydygier Medical University in Bydgoszcz: Technology of eye drops containing aloe (<u>Aloe arborescens</u> Mill.—Liliaceae) and eye drops containing both aloe and neomycin sulphate. Acta Poloniae Pharmaceutics. 60(1):31-9, 2003 Jan-Feb.

Koike, T., Beppu, H., Kuzuya, H., Maruta, K., Shimpo, K., Suzuki, M., Titani, K., Fujita, K.: A 35 kDa mannose-binding lectin with hemag-glutinating and mitogenic activities from 'Kidachi Aloe' (<u>Aloe arborescens</u> Miller var. natalensis Berger). Journal of Biochemistry 118, 1205-1210, 1995.

Koo, M.: Aloe vera: anticancer and antidiabetic effects. Phytother Res 8:461-4, 1994.

Kuo, P.L., Lin, T.C., Lin, C.C.: The antiproliferative activity of aloe-emodin is through p53-dependent and p21-dependent apoptotic pathway in human hepatoma cell lines. Life Sciences 71(16): 1879-1892, 2002.

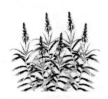

Kupchan, S.M., Karim, A.: Tumor inhibitors. 114. Aloe emodin: antileukemic principle isolated from Rhamnus frangula L.A systematic fractionation of an ethanol-water (1:1) extract of the seeds of Rhamnus frangula L., guided by assays for tumore-inhibitory activity, led to the isolation of aloe emodin (1). This compound was found to show significant antileukemic activity against the P-388 lymphocytic leuke-mia in mice. A noteworthy vehicle-dependence of the testing results is reported. In the light of this vehicle-dependence, the re-examination of other anthraquinone derivatives is recommended.

Lee, K.H., Hong, H.S., Lee, C.H., Kim, G.A.: Induction of apoptosis in human leukaemic cell lines K562, HL 60 and U9337 by diethylhexylphthlatate isolated from Aloe vera Linne. Journal of Pharmacy and Pharmacology 52(8):1037-1041, 2000.

Lee, K.H., KIim, J.H., Liu, D.S., Kim, C.H.: Anti-leukaemic and anti-mutagenic effects of di(2-ethylhexyl)phthalate isolated from Aloe vera Linne. Journal of Pharmacy and Pharmacology 52(5):593-598, 2000.

Lee, M.J., Yoon, S.H., Lee, S.K., Chung, M.H., Park, Y.I., Sung, C.K., Choi, J.S., Kim, K.W.: In vivo angiogenic activity of dichloromethane extracts of Aloe vera gel. Archives of Pharmacological Research. 18, 332-335, 1995.

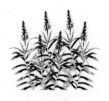

Lefkowitz, D., et al.: Effects of a glyconutrient on macrophage functions, International Journal of Immunopharmacology 22(4):299-308, 2000 Apr.

Leung, M.Y., Liu, C., Zhu, L.F., Hui, Y.Z., Yu, B., Fung, K.P.: Chemical and biological characterization of a polysaccharide biological response modifier from Aloe vera L. Glycobiology 14(6):501-5 10, 2004.

Lian, L.H., Park, E.J., Piao, H.S., Zhao, Y.Z., Soho, D.H.: Aloe-emodin-induced apoptosis in t-HSC/CI-6 cells involves a mitochondria-mediated pathway. Basic and Clinical Pharmacology and Toxicology 96(6):495-502, 2005.

Lin, J.G., Chen, G.W., Li, T.M., Chouh, S.T., Tan, T.W., Chung, J.G.: Aloe-emodin induces apoptosis in T24 human bladder cancer cells through the p53-dependent apoptotic pathway. Journal of Urology 175(1):343-347, 2006.

Lindblad, W.J., Thul, J.: Sustained increase in collagen biosynthesis in acemannan impregnated PVA implants in the rat. Wound Repair and Regeneration 2, 84, 1994.

Lissoni, P., Giani, L., Zerbini, S., Trabattoni, P., Rovelli, F., Division of Radiation Oncology, San Gerardo Hospital, Monza, Milan, Italy. Biotherapy with the pineal immuno-modulating hormone melatonin versus melatonin plus aloe vera in untreatable advanced solid neoplasms.

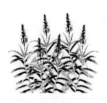

Liu, Y., Yang, H., Takatsuki, H., Sakanishi, A.: Effect of ultrasonic exposure of Ca++ -ATPase activity in plasma membrane from <u>Aloe arborescens</u> callus cells. Ultrasonic Sonochemistry 13(3):232-236, 2006.

Lorenzetti, L.J., Salisbury, R., Beal, J.L., Baldwin, J.N.: Bacterio-static properties of Aloe vera. Journal of Pharmaceutical Science 53, 1287, 1964.

Marshall, G.D., Druck, J.P.: In vitro stimulation of NK activity by acemannan. Journal of Immunology 150, 241A, 1993.

McDaniel. H.R., Pulse, T.: Predition and Results Obtained Using Oral Acemannan in 41 Symptomatic HIV Patients. IV International Conference on Aids, Stockholm, Sweden, June 12-16, 1988.

McDaniel, H. Reg., M.D.: Cancer, Is There A Role for Dietary Supplementation in Combination with Standard Cancer Therapy. Comprehensive Cancer Conference 2000, The Center for Mind-Body Medicine Washington, DC June 9-11, 2000 Sponsors: The University of Texas-Houston Medical School, The National Cancer Institute, The National Center for Complementary and Alternative Medicine, 2000.

McDaniel, H. Reg., M.D.: The Micronutrient Best Case Cancer Series: A Compendium of Medical Presentations Made at Cancer Conferences Between 2000 and 2004 documenting that the Quality of Life and Response to Standard Treatment

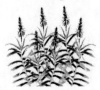

Protocols for Malignancy Improved with Dietary Supplementation. These conferences included: The Comprehensive Cancer 2003 Conference held in Washington, D.C. and sponsored by the Center for Mind Body Medicine, National Cancer Institute, National Center for Complementary and Alternative Medicine of the National Institutes of Health, First International Conference for Integrative Oncology held in New York City, NY, in November 2004 and sponsored by the National Center for Complementary and Alternative Medicine of the National Institutes of Health and the Society for Integrative Oncology, 2000-2004.

McDaniel, H. Reg., M.D.: Hepatitis General Antiviral Activity is Supported by Glyconutrient Dietary Supplementation. Hepatitis Conference 2000 Miami Beach, Florida, June 3-4, 2000.

McDaniel, H. Reg., M.D.: AIDS Patient Responses Validate in Vitro Experiments Indicating Micronutrient Dietary Supplementation (DS) Supports Innate Antiviral Mechanisms and Restores Immune Function. 9th World Congress on Clinical Nutrition, The University of Westminster, London, England, June 24-26, 2002.

McDaniel, H. Reg., M.D.: The Molecular Biology of How Dietary Supplements Support Optimal Human Health, Fisher Institute Vol 2, No. 3, April 2002

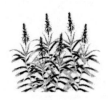

McDaniel, H. Reg., M.D.: Lymphocyte Levels in Acemannan Treated HIV-1 Infected Long-Term Survivors, Abstract # PO-B29-2179, IXth International Conf. on AIDS, Berlin, 1993.

McDaniel, H. Reg., M.D.: The Influence of Micronutrition in Combination with Standard Cancer Therapy on Malignacies: NCI Best Case Series. 1st Int. Conf. Interative Oncology, New York, NY, November, 2004.

McDaniel, H. Reg., M.D.: The Source of the Master Glyco-nutrient, Abstract International Aloe Science Council.

McDaniel, H. Reg., M.D.: Glyconutrition in Alzheimers's Disease: a pilot clinical survey, 1st Glycomics International Conference , Endowment for Medical Research, October 2005, Houston, TX.

McDaniel, H. Reg., M.D.: Response of Alzheimer's Disease to extended micronutrition, 2nd Glycomics International Conference, Endowment for Medical Research, October 2006, Houston, TX.

McDaniel, H. Reg., M.D.: A new horizon in optimal health and restoring health through use of nutraceuticals and herbs offers an unparalleled professional opportunity to health professionals, Washington, State Pharmaceutical Association, British Columbia, Jan.14-16, 2000.

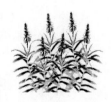

McDaniel, H. Reg., M.D. : The Impact of Glyconutrients on the Immune Function, Conference on Innate Immune Defense, Defense Threat Reduction Agency-DOD, Lansdowne, Virginia, September 2005

Merzlyak, M., Solovchenko, A., Pogosyan, S.: Department of Physiology of Microorganisms, Faculty of Biology, Moscow State University, 1 19992, GSP-2, Moscow, Russia. mnm@6. Celllmm.bio.msu.ru Optical properties of rhodoxanthin accumulated in <u>Aloe arborescens</u> Mill. Leaves under high-light stress with special reference to its photoprotective function. Photochemical & Photobiological Sciences. 4(4): 333-40, 2005 Apr.

Morita, H.; Mizuuchi, Y.; Abe, T.; Kohno, T.; Noguchi, H.; Abe, I.: Institution Mitsubishi Kagaku Institute of Life Sciences (MITILS). Cloning and functional analysis of novel aldo-keto reductase from <u>Aloe arborescens</u>. Biological 8, Pharmaceutical Bulletin. 30 (12):2262-7, 2007 Dec.

Nakasugi, Tohru; Komai, Koichiro Res. Lab. Med, Prod. Plant Origin Kinki Daigaku Nogakubu Kiyo (1994), 27, 47-54. An antimutagen from <u>Aloe Arborescens</u> Mill was isolated and identified. Methanol exts. from dried leaves of A. arborescens inhibited frameshift mutation induced by 3-amino-1-methyl-5H-pyrido [4, 3b] indole in Salmonella typhimurium TA98. The antimutagen isolated from the methanol exts. was identified as the anthraquinone Aloe-emodin. Aloe-emodin

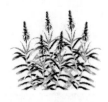

inhibited frameshift mutation by 60.3% at 0.1 mM/plate and 86.3% at 1.0 mM/plate whereas barbaloin, monoglucoside of Aloe-emodin, did not. Fresh A. aborescens leaves contained 1.17 ug/g (wet wt.) of Aloe-emodin. Aloe-emodin was also detected in A. ferox, A. vera, A. eru, and A. compacta by HPLC. These Aloe species may have substances that are useful for prevention of some forms of cancer.

Norikura, T., Kennedt, D.O., Nyarko, A.K., Kojima, A., Matsui, I.: Protective effect of aloe extract against the cytotoxicity of 1,4-naphthoquinone in isolated rat hepatocytes involves modulation in cellular thiol levels. Pharmacology & Toxicology 90(5):278-284, 2002.

Obata, M., Ito, S., Beppu, H., Fujita, K., Nagatsu, T.: Mechanism of anti-inflammatory and antithermal burn action of <u>Aloe arborescens</u> Miller var. Natalensis Berger. Phytotherapy Research 7, s30-s33, 1993.

Parish, Christopher R.: Innate Immune Mechanisms: Nonself Recognition, Australian National University, Canberra, Australia, July 1999.

Payne, J., Tissue Response to Aloe Vera Gel Following Periodontal Surgery, Thesis, Baylor University, 1970

Pecere, T., Gazzolz, M.V., Mucignat, C., Paralin, C., Vecchia, F. D., Cavaggioni, A., Pierce, R.F.: Comparison between the nutritional contents of the Aloe gel from conventionally and hydroponically grown plants. Erde International 1, 37-38, 1983.

Pecere, T., Gazzolz, M.V., Mucignat, C., Paralin, C., Vecchia, F. D., Cavaggioni, A., Basso, G., Diaspro, A., Salvato, B., Carli, M., Palu, G.: Aloe-emodin is a new type of anticancer agent with selective activity against neuroectodermal tumors. Cancer Research 60 (11):2800-2804, 2000.

Peuser, Michael: Capillaries Determine Our Fate/Aloe Empress of the Medical Plants, by St. Hubertus Produtos Naturals Ltda. Brazil: 91-101, 2003.

Pittman, J.C.: Immune-Enhancing Effects of Aloe, Health Conscious, 13(1) 28-30, 1992.

Pittman, John C.: Digestion and the Immune System and Aloe Vera Mucopolysaccharides.

Plaskett, Lawrance G. (BA, PhD, CChem, FRIC): Aloe vera and the human immune system. Aloe Vera Information Services (newsletter). Camelford, Cornwall, UK: Biomedical Information Services Ltd. Abstract: Specialized molecules in Aloe vera whole leaf extract interact with some special "receptor" substances that are embedded into the outer membrane of our immune system cells. The result is that the immune system cells are galvanized into action. In particular, the class of cells known as "phagocytes" increase the activities by which they attack and then engulf bacteria, waste products and debris. This increase in scavenging activities cleanses and protects the body, with knock-on benefits for a whole cascade of different medical conditions. The literature indicates that a common mechanism in this respect probably exists in both humans and animals and that both can benefit enormously from the use of Aloe vera, 1996, April.

Plaskett, Lawrance G. (BA, PhD, CChem, FRIC): Aloe vera and cancer. Aloe Vera Information Services (newsletter). Camelford, Cornwall, UK: Biomedical Information Services Ltd., 1996, September.

Plaskett, Lawrance, BA, PhD, CChem, FRIC: Aloe Vera, Aloe In Alternative Medicine Practice.

Plaskett, Lawrance G. (BA, PhD, CChem, FRIC): The healing properties of Aloe. *Aloe Vera Information Services* (newsletter). Camelford, Cornwall, UK: Biomedical Information Services Ltd., 1996, July.

Pugh, N., Ross, S.A., El Sohly, M.A., Pasca, D.S.: Characterization of *Aloeride, a new high-molecular weight polysaccharide from Aloe vera with potent immuno-stimulatory activity. Journal of Agricultural and Food Chemistry 49(2): 1030-1034, 2001.

Pulse, T.L. (MD), & Uhlig, Elizabeth (RRA): A significant improvement in a clinical pilot study utilizing nutritional supplements, essential fatty acids and stabilized Aloe vera juice in 29 HIV seropositive, ARC and AIDS patients. Journal of Advancement in Medicine, 3(4), 1990, Winter.

Qiu, Z., Jones, K., Wylie, M., Jia, G., Orndoref, S.: Modified Aloe barbadensis polysaccharide with immuno-regulating activity. Planta Medica 66(2): 152-156, 2000.

Reynolds, T., Dweck, A. C.: Aloe vera leaf gel: a review update. Journal of Ethnopharmacology. 68, 3-37, 1999.

Ross, S.A., El Sohly, M.A., Wilkins, S.P.: Quantitative analysis of Aloe vera mucilagenous polysaccharides in commercial Aloe vera products. Journal of AOAC International 80, 455-457, 1997.

Rubel, B.L.: Possible mechanisms of the healing actions of Aloe gel. Cosmetics and Toiletries 98, 109-114, 1983.

Sabeh, F., Wright, T., Norton, S.J.: Isozymes of superoxide dismutase from Aloe vera. Enzyme Protein 49, 212-221, 1996.

Saito, H.: Purification of active substances of <u>Aloe arborescens</u> Miller and their biological and pharmacological activity. Phytotherapy Research 7, S14-S19, 1993, 7 (Spec. Issue, Proceedings of the International Congress of Phytotherapy, 1991), S14-S19. The authors purified Aloctin A from <u>Aloe arborescens</u> Miller and defined its chem., biol. and pharmacol. activities. Aloctin A consists of two discrete bands, a and b, with a combined S-S bond. Its mol. wt. for "a" is 7500 and

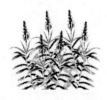

the mol. wt. for "b" is 10,500. Aloctin A has many biol. and pharmacol. activities as follows: 1. hemag-glutinating activity; 2. cytoagglutinating activity; 3. mito-genic activity of lymphocytes; 4. ppt. – forming reactivity with a2-macroglobulin; 5. complement C3 activating acti-vity; 6. inhibition of heat-induced hemolysis of rat erythro-cytes; 7. anti-tumor effect; 8. anti-inflammatory effect; 9. inhibition of gastric secretion and gastric lesions.

Saito, H.: Aloe's Effectiveness As An Anti-Inflammatory Agent, Department of Pharmacy Aichi Cancer Center, Nagoya, Japan

Sampedro, M.C., Artola, R.L., Murature, M., Murature, D., Ditamo, Y., Roth, G.A., Kivatinitz, S.: Mannan from Aloe saponaria inhibits tumoral cell activation and proliferation. International Immuno-pharmacology 4(3):4 1 1-4 18, 2004.

Saoo, K., Miki, H., Ohmori, M., Winters, W.D.: Antiviral activity of Aloe extracts against cytomegalovirus. Phytotherapy Research 10, 348-350, 1996.

Schechter, S.R.: Aloe vera: the healing plant. Health Foods Business, 23-24, 1994.

Shelton, R.M.: Aloe vera: Its chemical and therapeutic proper-ties. International Journal of Dermatology 30, 679-683, 1991.

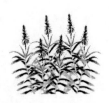

Shida, T., Yagi, A., Nishimura, H., Nishioka, I.: Effect of Aloe extract on peripheral phagocytosis in adult bronchial asthma. Planta medica 51, 273-275, 1985.

Shimpo, K., Beppu, H., Chihara, T., Kaneko, T., Shinzato, M., Sonoda, S.: Fujita Memorial Nanakuri Institute, Fujita Health University, Tsu, 1865 Isshiki-cho, Hisai Mie 514-1296 Japan. Effects of <u>Aloe arborescens</u> ingestion on azoxymethane-induced intestinal carcinogenesis and hematological and bio-chemical parameters of male F344 rats. Asian Pacific Journal of Cancer Prevention: Apjcp. 7(4):585-90, 2006 Oct-Dec.

Shimpo, K., Chihara, T., Beppu, H., Ida, C., Kaneko, T., Nagatsu, T., Kuzuya, H.: Inhibition of azoxymethane-induced aberrant crypt foci formation in rat colorectum by whole leaf <u>Aloe arborescens</u> Miller, var. natalensis Berger. Phytotherapy Research 15(8):705-711, 2001.

Shimpo, K., Ida, C., Chihara, T., Beppu, H., Kaneko, T., Kuzuya, H.: <u>Aloe arborescens</u> extract inhibits TPA-induced ear oedema, putrescine increase and tumour promotion in mouse skin. Phytotherapy Research 16(5):491-493, 2002.

Shimpo, K., Chihara, T., Beppu, H., Ida, C., Kaneko, T., Hoshino, M., Kuzuya, H.: Inhibition of azoxymethane-induced DNA adduct formation by <u>Aloe arborescens</u> var. natalensis. Asian Pacific Journal of Cancer Prevention 4(3):247-251, 2003.

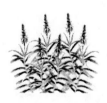

Siegel, Dr. R., M.D.: Aloe, Immunity and Health CareScience papers presented to the Annual International Environmental Conference, 1998.

Siegel, Dr. R., M.D.: The Science of Immunity/The Regulation of Immunity

Siegel, Dr. R., M.D.: Natural Plant Molecules.

Soeda, M., Otomo, M., Ome, M., Kawashima, K.: Studies on antibacterial and anti-fungal activity of Cape Aloe. Nippon Saikingaku Zasshi 21, 609-614, 1966.

Stuart, R.W., Lefkowitz, D.L., Lincoln, J.A., Howard, K., Gelderman, M.P., Lefkowitz, S.S.: Upregulation of phagocytosis and candicidal activity of macrophages exposed to the immunostimulant, acemannan. International Journal of Immunopharmacology 19, 75-82, 1997.

Suga, Takayuki and Hirata, Toshifumi: The Efficacy of the Aloe Plant's Chemical Constituents and Biological Activities, Department of Chemistry, Faculty of Science Hiroshima University, Higashisnda-machi, Naka-ku, Allured Publishing Corp.Hiroshima. Japan, 1983

Sydiskis, R.J., Owen, D.G., Lohr, J.L., Rosler, K.H., Blomster, R.N.: Inactivation of enveloped viruses by anthraquinones extracted from plants. Antimicrobial Agents and Chemotherapy 35, 2463-2466, 1991.

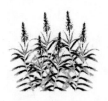

Syed, T.A., Ahmad, A., Holt, A.H., Ahmad, S.A., Ahmad, S.H., Afzal, M.: Management of psoriasis with Aloe vera extract in a hydrophilic cream: a placebo-controlled, double blind study. Tropical Medicine and International Health 1, 505-509, 1996.

T'Hart, L.A., Nibbering, P.H., van den Barselaar, M.T., van Dijk, H., van den Berg, A.J., Labadie, R.P.: Effects of low molecular constituents from Aloe vera gel on oxidative metabolism and cytotoxic and bactericidal activities of human neutrophils. International Journal for Immunopharmacology 12, 427-434, 1990.

T'Hart, L.A., van den Berg, A. J. J., Kuis, L., van Dijk, H., Labadie, R.P.: An anti-complementary polysaccharide with immuno-logical adjuvant activity from the leaf parenchyma gel of Aloe vera. Planta Medica 55, 509-512, 1989.

T'Hart, L.A., van Enckevort, P.H., van Dijk, H., Zaat, R., de Silva, K.T.D., Labadie, R.P.: Two functionally and chemically distinct immunomodulatory compounds in the gel of Aloe vera. Journal of Ethnopharmacology 23, 61-71, 1988.

Tanaka, M., Misawa, E., Ito, Y., Habara, N., Nomaguchi, K., Yamada, M., Toida, T., Hayasawa, H., Takase, M., Inagaki, M., Higuchi, R., Biochemical Research Laboratory, Morinaga Milk Industry Co., Ltd, Kanagawa, Japan: Identification of five

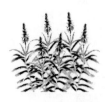

phytosterols from Aloe vera gel as anti-diabetic compounds. Biological 8, Pharmaceutical Bulletin. 29(7):1418-22, 2006 Jul.

Teradaira, R., Shinzato, M., Beppu, H., Fujita, K.: Antigastric ulcer effects of <u>Aloe arborescens</u> Mill. var. natalensis Berger. Phytotherapy Research 7, S34-S36, 1993.

Tizard, I., Carpenter, R.H., Kemp, M.: Immunoregulatory effects of a cytokine release enhancer (Acemannan). International Congress of Phytotherapy, 1991, Seoul, Korea, 68, 1991.

Tizard, Ian R., BVMS, PhD, Carpenter, Robert H., DVM, MS, McAnalley, Bill H., PhD, and Kemp, Maurice C.: The biological activities of mannans and related complex carbohydrates. Department of Veterinary Microbiology and Parasitology, College of Veterinary Medicine. Texas A&M University, College Station, TX, and Carrington Laboratories, Inc. Irving, TX, USA August 21, 1989.

Tizard, I.; Kemp, M., ScienceDirect-International Immuno-pharmacology, Mannan from Aloe saponaria inhibits tumoral cell activation and proliferation, International Immunopharmacology Volume 4, Issue 3, March 2004, Pages 411-418. Research by immunologist Ian Tizard, Ph.D. and virologist Maurice Kemp, Ph.D. from Texas A&M led to the discovery that Aloe mucopolysaccharide is taken into a special leukocyte, the macrophage, and this cell is stimulated to release messenger molecules called cytokines (interferons, inter-

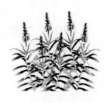

leukines, prostaglandins, tumor necrosis factor and stem-cell growth factors.) Tumors release a chemical that attracts blood circulation so that malignant cells have a supply to the tumor and it therefore dies. All of the immune modulating effects from Aloe contribute greatly to the prevention and healing of malignant cells.

Vinson, J.A., Al Kharrat, H., Andreoli, L.: Effect of Aloe vera preparations on the human bioavailability of vitamins C and E. Department of Chemistry, University of Scranton, Scranton, PA, 18510 4626, USA. Received 18 July 2003; accepted 19 December 2003

Wang, Z.W., Zhopu, J.M., Huang, Z.S., Yang, A.P., Liu, Z.L., Xia, Y.F., Zeng, Y.X., Zhu, X.F.: Aloe polysaccharide mediated radio-protective effect through the inhibition of apoptosis. Journal of Radiation Research (Tokyo) 45(3):447-454, 2004.

Wasserman, L., Avigad, S., Berry, E., Nordenberg, J., Fenig, E.: The effect of aloe-emodin on the proliferation of a new merkel carcinoma cell line. American Journal of Dermatopathology 24(1): 17-22, 2002.

Wickline, M.M.: Prevention and treatment of acute radiation dermatitis: a literature review. Oncology Nursing Forum 3 1(2):237-247, 2004.

Willner, Robert E., M.D., Ph.D.: Whole Leaf Aloe Vera: The Cancer Solution, Peltec Publishing Co., Inc., 1994.

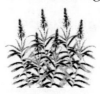

Winters, W.D.: Immunoreactive Lectins in Leaf Gel from Aloe barbadensis Miller, Phytoherapy Research. Vol. 7, S23-S25 (1993)

Winters, Wendell D.: Aloe Medicinal Substances Present And Future Potentials, Associate Professor of Microbiology Director, Phytobiology Studies Program, University of Texas Health Science Center, Polypeptides of Aloe barbadensis Miller., Phytotherapy Research, February, 2006.

Winters, W.D.: Aloemannan, Significant Antitumor Efficacy, Health Science Center, University Of Texas, 1977. In 1977, while conducting a series of animal experiments using aloemannan (a mucopolysaccharide of <u>Aloe arborescens</u>), detected aloemannan, a significant antitumor efficacy. Unlike usual anticancer drugs killing cancer cells directly, it acts as a stimulus for the body's defense mechanism, or immunity to suppress tumor. In other words, it prohibits multiplication of cancer cells while it is coexistent with them. Prof. Winters and his group of the Health Science Center at the University of Texas verified their test-tube experiments using human cervical cancer cells that Aloe vera extract prohibits the growth of cancer cells.

Wozniewski, T., Blaschek, W., Franz, G.: Isolation and structure analysis of a glucomannan from the leaves of <u>Aloe arborescens</u> var. Miller. Carbohydrate Research 198, 387-391, 1990.

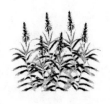

Yagi, A., Harada, N., Shimomura, K., Nishioka, I.: Bradykinin-degrading glycoprotein in <u>Aloe arborescens</u> var. natalensis. Planta Medica 53, 19-21, 1987.

Yagi, A., Harada, N., Yamada, H., Iwadare, S., Nishioka, I.: Anti-bradykinin active material in Aloe saponaria. Journal of Pharmaceutical Sciences 71, 1172-1174, 1982.

Yagi, A., Shida, T., Nishimura, H.: Effect of amino acids in Aloe extract on phagocytosis by peripheral neutrophil in adult bronchial asthma. Japanese Journal of Allergology 36, 1094-1101, 1987.

Yamamoto, M., Masui, T., Sugiyama, K., Yokota, M., Nakagomi, K., Nakazawa, H.: Anti-inflammatory active constituents of <u>Aloe arborescens</u> Miller. Agricultural and Biological Chemistry 55, 1627-1629, 1991.

Yoshimoto, R.; Kondoh, N.; Isawa, M.; Hamuro, J.: Plant Lectin, ATF1011, On The Tumor Cell Surface Augments Tumor-Specific Immunity Through Activation Of T Cells Specific For The Lectin. Cancer Immunol Immunother 25(1):25-30 1987. The possibility that a plant lectin as a carrier protein would specifically activate T cells, resulting in the augmentation of anti-tumor immunity was investigated. ATF1011, a nonmito-genic lectin for T cells purified from <u>Aloe arborescens</u> Mill, bound equally to normal and tumor cells.

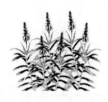

Glossary

Aloe-emodin: A noval antitumor chemotherapeutic agent. A substance found in certain plants, including Aloe arborescens and Aloe vera. It belongs to a family of compounds called anthraquinones, which have shown anti-inflammatory and anti-cancer effects.

Alzheimer's disease (AD): the most common form of dementia. This incurable, degenerative and terminal disease was first described by German psychiatrist Alöis Alzheimer in 1901. Generally it is diagnosed in people over 65 years of age, although the less-prevalent early-onset Alzheimer's can occur much earlier. The cause and progresssion of Alzheimer's disease are not well understood. Research indicates that the disease is associated with plaques and tangles in the brain. As the disease advances, symptoms include confusion, irritability and aggression, mood swings, language breakdown, long-term memory loss, and the general withdrawal of the sufferer as his or her senses decline. Gradually, minor and major bodily functions are lost, ultimately leading to death. The mean life expectancy following diagnosis is approximately seven years.

Antiophidic serum: Anti-venom serum.

Aqueous humour: Thick watery substance that fills the space between the lens and the cornea.

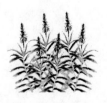

Arthritis: A disease reaction and a symptom of a disease. It is an inflammation caused by crystallized toxic waste from a diet of constipating foods and/or synthetic chemicals that reduce moisture in the joints and cause waste deposits in the joints. The presence of arthritis can mean that the body is not dissolving and flushing out toxins or minerals. The waste deposits can collect and congest in the tissues and muscles. The body immobilizes (stops) any part of the body that needs repairs. For example, a sprained wrist becomes stiff and a strained muscle becomes stiff (called nature's cast). An injured part of the body remains sore or stiff until it is repaired. If repairs are not made, that part becomes permanently stiff (calcified) or immobilized. The crystallized waste in impaired or immobilized joints and/or tissue can rub against each other causing inflammation. Arthritis is inflammation caused by waste in the bone joints while rheumatism is waste in the muscles. The body uses heat (inflammation) to increase circulation, kill bacteria and bring healing nutrients to arthritic areas.

Ascomycetes: Class of fungi characterized by the presence of asci and ascospores.

Basidiomycetes: Class of true fungi that produce their spores at the tips of swollen hyphae.

Bilirubin: Substance formed when red blood cells are broken down.

Blennorrhea: Free discharge from mucous surfaces.

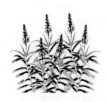

Cancer: The word Cancer means crab and/or creeping sore. Cancer tissue and cells cover a broad spectrum of malignant (bad) neoplasms (new cells). There are over one hundred types of bad new cells (malignant neoplasms) classified as cancer. Each is believed to have a different cause. The types of cancer are _carcinomas,_ which affect glands, skin, organs, and mucous membrane skin; _lymphomas,_ which affect lymph glands and fluid; _sarcomas,_ which affect bones, muscles, connective tissue; and _leukemia,_ which affect blood.

Cancer develops when cells in a part of the body begin to grow out of control. Although there are many kinds of cancer, they all start because of out-of-control growth of abnormal cells.

Normal body cells grow, divide, and die in an orderly fashion. During the early years of a person's life, normal cells divide more rapidly until the person becomes an adult. After that, cells in most parts of the body divide only to replace worn-out or dying cells and to repair injuries.

Because cancer cells continue to grow and divide, they are different from normal cells. Instead of dying, they outlive normal cells and continue to form new abnormal cells.

Cancer cells often travel to other parts of the body where they begin to grow and replace normal tissue. The cancer cells get into the bloodstream or lymph vessels of our body. When cells from a cancer like breast cancer spread to another organ like the liver, the cancer is still called breast cancer, not liver cancer.

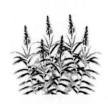

Cancer cells develop because of damage to DNA. This substance is in every cell and directs all its activities. Most of the time when DNA becomes damaged the body is able to repair it. In cancer cells, the damaged DNA is not repaired. People can inherit damaged DNA, which accounts for inherited cancers. Many times though, a person's DNA becomes damaged from exposure to something in the environment, like cigarette smoke.

Cancer usually forms as a solid tumor. Some cancers, like leukemia, do not form tumors. Instead, these cancer cells involve the blood and blood-forming organs and circulate to other tissues where they grow.

Not all tumors are cancerous. Benign (non-cancerous) tumors do not spread to other parts of the body (metastasize) and, with very rare exceptions, are not life-threatening.

Different types of cancer can behave very differently. For example, lung cancer and breast cancer are very different diseases. They grow at different rates and respond to different treatments.

Carbuncle: Painful localized bacterial infection of the skin and subcutaneous tissue that usually has several openings through which pus is discharged.

Coronary Heart Disease (CHD): CHD is caused by a thickening of the inside walls of the coronary arteries. This thickening, called atherosclerosis narrows the space through which blood can flow, decreasing and sometimes completely cutting off the

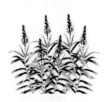

supply of oxygen and nutrients to the heart. It is usually caused by a combination of non-holistic practices such as poor nutrition, environmental pollution, destructive eating habits and deterioration of the body. Many other factors can cause this disease reaction such as high and low blood pressure, acid ash, fat deposits, thermal glandular fatigue and loss of vein and artery flexibility.

Atherosclerosis usually occurs when a person has high levels of cholesterol, a fat-like substance in the blood. Cholesterol and fat circulating in the blood build up on the walls of the arteries. This build-up narrows the arteries and can slow or block the flow of blood. When the level of cholesterol in the blood is high, there is a greater chance that it will be deposited onto the artery walls. This process begins in most people during childhood and the teenage years, and worsens as they get older.

In addition to high blood cholesterol, high blood pressure and smoking also contribute to CHD. On the average, each of these doubles your chance of developing heart disease. Therefore, a person who has all three risk factors is eight times more likely to develop heart disease than someone who has none. Obesity and physical inactivity are other factors that can lead to CHD. Being overweight increases the likelihood of developing high blood cholesterol and high blood pressure while physical inactivity increases the risk of heart attack. Regular exercise, good nutrition and smoking cessation are key to controlling the risk factors for CHD.

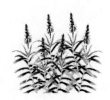

Cryptococcus: Tiny yeast-like fungus.

Cytomegalovirus (CMV): Type of virus that can cause inapparant infections in healthy individuals but is dangerous to immunosuppressed patients; a member of the herpes family of viruses.

Cytomycosis: Fungal disease that may result in flu-like symptoms

Dermatitis: Inflammation of the skin.

Diabetes: A disease of the pancreas. The melanin centers of the pancreas (Islet of Langerhaus) are harmed or damaged. The condition exists when the body has sugar (natural fuel for the body) available, but fails to recognize it. This causes excess sugar to accumulate, which the body gets rid of by excess urination. The urine will become morbid and change in odor and color. Excessive urinating causes thirst, dehydration, weight loss, loss of appetite, and an overworked kidney and pancreas. The pancreas secretes the hormone insulin, which stimulates the use of sugar. Diseases, emotions and /or social stressors can over stimulate the pituitary and/or adrenals, which overtaxes the pancreas, resulting in diabetes. People can have misdiagnosed or subclinical diabetes-related diseases of high blood pressure, hyperactivity, kidney failure, cataracts, nerve damage, glaucoma, infertility, mood swings, hair loss, bone loss, etc. Diabetes is usually caused by overeating and refined carbohydrates (bleached white flour, white rice, white grits, cooked white potatoes, and refined white sugar). Eating

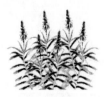

excessive amounts of animal flesh and cooked animal fats (fats and proteins change to sugar in the body) can cause diabetes.

Dysphoria: Abnormal depression and discontent.

Dyspnea: Difficult, painful breathing or shortness of breath.

Ectogenous: Originating from or due to influences from outside of the organism.

Endocardium: Thin serous membrane, composed of endothelial tissue, that lines the interior of the heart.

Endogenous: Developing or originating within the organism or arising from causes within the organism.

Epithelial: Refers to the cells that line the internal and external surfaces of the body.

Epithelium: The outermost layer of cells of the cornea and the eye's first defense against infection.

Eructation: Expelling air from the stomach through the mouth.

Erythema: Reddening of the skin.

Erythematous: Redness of the skin caused by capillary congestion.

Exanthematous: Refers to any eruptive disease or fever.

Excrescences: Abnormal outgrowths or enlargements of some part of the body.

Exudation: Slow escape of liquids from blood vessels through pores or breaks in the cell membranes.

Fibroblast: A connective tissue cell that makes and secretes collagen proteins.

Fungi Imperfecti: A phylum of fungi in which sexual reproduction is not known or in which one of the mating types has not yet been discovered.

Glycobiology: Refers to a relatively new field of science that looks at saccharide compounds and how they impact health. Research into glyconutrients reveals a multi-faceted subject that studies the diverse effects of sugars on cellular functions and disease. — Elkins, Rita, M.H.: *Miracle Sugars, The Glyconutrient Link to Disease Prevention and Improved Health*, Woodland Publishing, 2003

Glyconutrients: Beneficial plant sugars, a biochemical that contains a sugar molecule. Certain plant parts contain glyconutrients. A common source is Aloe vera and Aloe arborescens. Chemists now believe eight dietary sugars (also called saccharides, plant sugars or carbohydrates) play a profound role in the maintenance of human health. Unlike white sugar, these plant sugars contribute to cellular protection from microbial invaders and autoimmune syndromes.

Research over the last decade has revealed that sugars that coat cell surfaces (glycoforms) enable cells to talk to each other. When these sugars pair up with proteins, they form glycoproteins. When they combine with a fat molecule, a glycolipid is formed. Glycoproteins and glycolipids cover every cell in the body and serve as communication lines between cells. The

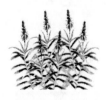

proper relay of information between cells determines your health status. Your immune cells cannot relay vital messages without these glycoforms, and your body cannot create enough glycoforms without sufficient levels of the essential eight glyconutrients, which are glucose, mannose, galatose, xylose, fucose, N-acetylglucosamine, N-acetylgalatosamine, and N-acetyl-neuraminic acid.

A great deal of scientific evidence suggests that consuming certain obscure plant sugars found in nature work to direct the action of the immune cells and can make the difference between optimal and mediocre immune function. Herbs like Aloe vera and Aloe arborescens, which are scientifically designated as powerful immune complements, are full of complex sugars called polysaccharides, which stimulate desirable immune activity. They contain two important sugars: glucomannan and mannose. Acetylated mannose, also known as acemannan, is a bioactive sugar component found in aloe that has been shown to be a powerful, effective immune support.

The essential eight glyconutrient sugars are engineered to instruct the immune system on where to go and what to kill in preventing a number of biological disorders. Consuming glyconutrients does not treat diseases directly but enables the body to optimize its own functions and systems that promote healing and protection from within. It does so at the cellular level, appearing to "recalibrate" cell to cell communication in the process of restoring balance. The higher the intake of glyconutrients, the more raw materials your body has to

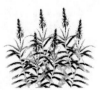

balance its immune cell networks. Therapeutic glyconutrient supplementation has become a means of bridging the gap between the ideal diet rich in a wide array of live plant food and the standard diet that is typically high in meat consumption while low in plants. — Elkins, Rita, M.H.: *Miracle Sugars, The Glyconutrient Link to Disease Prevention and Improved Health*, Woodland Publishing, 2003

Helminths: Parasitic worms.

Hemolytopoietic: Relating to the process of blood destruction and blood making.

Hemoptysis: Expectoration of blood from some part of the respiratory tract.

Homeostasis: The property of an open system, especially living organisms, to regulate its internal environment to maintain a stable, constant condition.

Hyperuricemia: Abnormally high level of uric acid in the blood.

Idiopathic: Arising from an obscure or unknown cause.

Imbricated: To overlap in a regular pattern.

Leukemia: (Greek leukos, "white;" aima, "blood") is a cancer of the blood or bone marrow and is characterized by an abnormal proliferation (production by multiplication) of blood cells, usually white blood cells (leukocytes). Leukemia is a broad term covering a spectrum of diseases. In turn, it is part of the even broader group of diseases called hematological neoplasms.

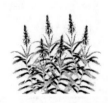

Lupus: How does it feel? Many people with lupus feel tired, experience joint aches and pains, loss of hair, or scarring skin lesions, while others may develop complications with involvement of the kidneys or central nervous system. The symptoms can be persistent or intermittent, and the devastating reality is that many women don't even know they have the disease. Lupus, an autoimmune disease in which antibodies react against the body's own tissue, affects nearly 250,000 Americans. The arthritis-related disease is a chronic and sometimes life-threatening disease that occurs in one of three forms: discoid lupus, which affects the skin; drug-induced lupus, which occurs because of a reaction to one or more drugs and usually disappears when the person stops taking the drug; and systemic lupus erythematosus (or SLE), which involves the skin, joints, kidneys, nervous system, lungs, heart and/or other organs.

Lymphoadenopathy: Abnormally enlarged lymph nodes. Commonly called "swollen glands."

Metastasize: To spread from one part of the body to another.

Moniliasis: Disease caused by the fungus Monilia; also known as Candidiasis (yeast infection).

Mucoid exudates: Serious nasal discharges.

Mycobacterium leprae: Bacterium that causes leprosy.

Myeloproliferative disorders: Group of conditions that cause an overproduction of blood cells (platelets, white blood cells, and red blood cells) in the bone marrow.

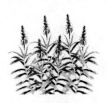

Myocardial Infarction: A heart attack.

Necrosis: The name given to unnatural death of cells and living tissue. It begins with cell swelling, chromatin digestion, and disruption of the plasma membrane and organelle membranes.

Osostomia: Bad breath.

Overweight/obesity: In some countries, a high percentage of adults are overweight or obese. Being overweight or obese increases the risk not only for heart disease, but also for other conditions, including stroke, gallbladder disease, arthritis, breast, colon and other cancers. Being overweight and obese are determined by two key measures — body mass index or BMI — and waist circumference. BMI relates height to weight.

Papule: Small solid rounded bump rising from the skin that is usually less than one centimeter in diameter.

Parenchyma: Functional parts of an organ.

Perturbation: Unhappy and worried mental state.

Phycomycetes: Group of fungi possessing hyphae that are usually nonseptate (without cross walls).

Polycythemia vera: Abnormal increase in blood cells (primarily red blood cells) due to excess production of the cells by the bone marrow.

Precordial: Pertaining to the region over the heart or stomach.

Protozoa: Single-celled organism.

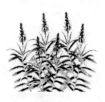

Pustule: Small collection of pus in the top layer of skin.

Putrefactive: Causing or promoting bacterial putrefaction.

Sebaceous glands: Normal gland of the skin that empties an oily secretion into the hair follicle near the surface of the skin.

Septicemia: Disease caused by the spread of bacteria and their toxins in the bloodstream; also called blood poisoning.

Sternocleidomastoid: One of the two muscles located on the front of the neck that serve to turn the head from side to side.

Streptococcal cellulitis: Spreading bacterial infection just below the skin surface caused by Streptococcus pyogenes.

Subendocardial ischemia: Insufficient blood supply to the area under the endocardium.

Synergism: The capacity of all the physical and chemical components of the plant to function together, in order to bring greater benefit than the benefit given by the single elements individually.

Thallophytes: Members of the lowest phylum of plants.

Tophaceous: Refers to deposits of crystallized monosodium urate in people with longstanding hyperuricemia.

Toxoplasmosis: Parasitic disease contracted through contact with infected undercooked meat.

Transudation: Passage of a fluid or solute through a membrane by a hydrostatic or osmotic pressure gradient.

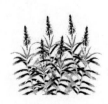

Tricuspid valve: Valve that separates the upper and lower chambers of the right side of the heart.

Tubular Necrosis: A kidney disorder involving damage to the tubule cells of the kidneys, resulting in acute kidney failure.

Urates: Uric acid deposits composed of salt crystals formed from uric acid.

Vesicant: Blistering agent.

Vesicles: Small fluid-filled blisters.

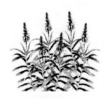

Index

1

10 days, 21

A

A Silent Cure, 33
Abscess, 63
Acemannan, 149, 151, 161
Acidity, 64
Acne, 65
Addiction, 65
Ahola, Robert, 33, 59
AIDS, 43, 66, 67, 138, 141, 150, 151, 156
Alcohol, 1, 24
Allergies, 68
Aloctin A, 145, 156
Aloe
    Myth-Magic-Medicine, 33
Aloe and the Sickness from A to Z, 60
Aloe arborescens, 7, 11, 15, 26, 27, 28,
    136, 142, 144, 145, 146, 149, 152,
    153, 156, 158, 161, 163, 164, 165,
    172, 173
Aloe Medicinal Substances, 163
Aloe ointment, 120
Aloe-based ointment, 111, 113
Aloe-based treatment, 59
Aloe-emodin, 135, 136, 148, 152, 154,
    165
Aloemannan, 163
Aloin, 37
Alzheimer's, 69, 70
Alzheimer's Disease, 69, 71, 151
Amazonian natives, 41

American Podiatric Medical, 140, 141
Anaplastic leukocytes, 112
Angioedema, 95
Anorexia, 71
Anthrax, 72
Anti-diabetic effects, 136
Anti-Inflammatory Agent, 144, 157
Anti-leukaemic, 147
Antitumor Effects of Aloe Vera, 139
Antitumor Efficacy, 163
Aphonia, 72
Arterial failure, 73
Arterial hypertension, 106
Arteriosclerosis, 74
Arthritis, 75, 166
Articulation (joint) pains, 98
Asthma, 75

B

Babosa, 3, 33, 61
Baldness, 77
Birthmarks, 77
Blisters, 78
Blood, 64
Boil, 101
Bonacin, Vilson Francesco, 61
Brazilian plant recipe, 7
Bronchitis, 78
Bruises, 79
Burns, 79
Bursitis, 80

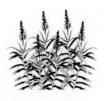

C

Cancer, 2, 7, 8, 26, 28, 33, 34, 35, 59, 81,
  82, 96, 136, 141, 142, 144, 149, 154,
  157, 158, 164, 167, 168
Cancer Can Be Cured!, 7, 8, 26, 28, 33,
  34, 35, 59, 82
Cancer Immunology Immuno-
  therapy, 141
Cancer Research, 136, 154
Candidiasis, 83, 175
Capillaries Determine Our Fate, 154
Carli, Professor Modesto, 81
Carrisyn, 68
Cataract, 83
Cavities, 99
Cellulitis, 85
CHD, 168, 169
Chemotherapy, 142
Chlamydia trachomatis, 126
Cirrhosis, 85
Coats, Bill C., 33
Cold, 86
Colic, 87
Colitis, 87
Commercial marketers, 26, 35
Complementary and Alternative
  Medicine, 150
Conductor-Orchestra Concept Of
  Aloe Vera, 140
Congestion, 88
Cook, Bill R., 33
Coronary Heart Disease, 168
Cough, 88
Cryptococcus, 66, 170
Cures, 1, 4, 59, 61, 81, 133
Cuts, 89

Cystitis, 89

D

Dandruff, 90
Danhof, Ivan E., 77
Dark containers, 20
Depression, 90, 91
Dermatitis, 91, 170
Diabetes, 92, 137, 141, 170
Digestion, 154
Discouragement, 93
Dislocations, 92
Distension, 94
Distillate, 18
Doses, 11
Drugs, 137
Dysentery, 94

E

Edema, 95, 141
Enteritis, 95
Epidermitis, 96
Epstein-Barr virus, 96
Eruption/Rash, 96
Erysipelas, 97
Exanthema, 97
Eye disease, 97

F

Fever, 52, 56, 99
Fissures, 99
Flatulence, 100
Franciscan style, 61
Fungus, 76, 100
Furuncle, 101

G

Gangrene, 101
Gastric hyperacidity, 64
Gel, 26, 153, 163
Gingivitis, 102
Glaucoma, 102
Glycobiology, 136, 148, 172
Glycomics, 151
Glyconutrient, 142, 150, 172, 174
Glyconutrients, 152, 172
Gout, 103

H

Halitosis, 103
Headaches, 98
Healing, 141, 145
Health Science Center at the
    University of Texas, 163
Hemorrhoids, 104
Hennessee, Odus M., 33
Hepatitis, 105, 150
Herpes, 96, 105, 131
Herpes simplex, 105
Herpes zoster, 105
Herpes-like virus, 96
HIV, 66, 149, 151, 156
HIV-1 Infected Long-Term Survivors,
    151
Hives, 128
Honey, 1, 17, 23, 92
Hypersensitivity, 68
Hypertension, 106

I

Immunopharmacology, 148, 160

Immuno-stimulating properties, 137
Indigestion, 107
Infection, 83, 96
Infections, 102, 107
Inflammation of the liver, 105
Ingrown toenails, 108
Insomnia, 108
Intestinal parasites, 108
Irritation of the mouth, 109
Itching, 109
Itching of any type, 109

J

Jaundice, 110

L

Laryngitis, 111
Leaf, 139, 163
Leaves, 152
Lecardonnel, Dr. Marie, 60
Leprosy, 111
Leukemia, 111, 174
Linus Pauling Institute of Science &
    Medicine, 136
Lupus, 112, 175
Lymphoadenopathy, 175
Lymphoma, 96

M

Malignacies, 151
Mastitis, 113
McDaniel, Reg, 68
Meningitis, 113
Migraine, 114
Molecular Biology, 150

Moscow State University, 152
Multiple sclerosis, 114
Muscle cramp, 115
Muscular aches, 98
Muscular distension, 94
Mycobacterium leprae, 111, 175
Myeloproliferative disorders, 175

N

National Center for Complementary
    and Alternative Medicine, 149, 150
National Institutes of Health and the
    Society for Integrative Oncology,
    150
Nausea, 116
Nausea of any type, 116
Necrosis, 101, 176, 178
New Guide to Aloe, 60
North Texas Research Laboratory, 139

O

Obesity, 117, 169
Odor, 117
Olympic Games, 93
Oncology, 148, 150, 151, 162
Optimal Human Health, 150
Oxidation, 69

P

Pain, 52, 55, 120, 141
Palu, Professor Giorgio, 81
Pancreatitis, 118
Peptic ulcer, 128
Phytotherapy, 137, 143, 144, 145, 153,
    156, 157, 158, 161, 163

Phytotherapy Research, 137, 143, 144,
    145, 153, 156, 157, 158, 163
Plant, 152, 159, 164
Preparation, 1, 11, 31
Presbyopia, 97, 116
Prostatitis, 119
Prostatitis/Prostatism, 119
Pseudo-tumor cerebri, 106
Psoriasis, 119
Pulmonary edema, 95
Pyrosis, 124

Q

Quality of life, 46

R

Radical-scavenging effect, 136
Recipe, 1, 5, 7, 11
Renovascular hypertension, 106

S

Sarcoma, 145
Sciatica, 120
Sebaceous glands, 177
Seborrhoea, 121
Sinusitis, 121
Sprain, 122
Standard Cancer Therapy, 149, 151
Sterility, 122
Stevens, Neil, 59, 61, 127
Stiff neck, 123
Stiff neck (Torticollis), 123
Stings, 123
Stomach aches, 98
Stomach acid, 124

Streptococcal cellulitis, 177
Synergism, 177

T

T lymphocytes, 66
Tendonitis, 125
Texas A&M University, 161
The Curative Power of Aloe, 59
The Silent Healer, 59
Tonsillitis, 125
Tooth aches, 98
Trachoma, 126
Treatment, 139, 149
Truth, 41
Tuberculosis, 126
Tumors, 162

U

Ulcer, 127
University of Padua, 81
University of Texas, 149, 163
University of Texas-Houston Medical
    School, 149

University of Westminster, London,
    England, 150
Urticaria, 128

V

Vaginitis, 129
Varix, 129
Vomiting, 52, 55

W

Weakness, 130
Weights and measurements, 1, 15
Whole Leaf Aloe Vera, 162
    The Cancer Solution, 162
Wound healing, 140
Wounds, 130, 141
Wounds of all types, 130

Z

Zoster, 131

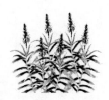